A BROKEN LIFE:

Drugs, Addiction, Why?

By

Patricia Sutton Burgess

This is the true story of the 48-year struggle of one young man as he lived it trying to fit into a niche of society while dealing with problems attributable to rape, mental illness and/or drug and alcohol addiction.

Printed by Create Space, An Amazon.com Company

ISBN: 13:978-1517344993

ISBN: 10-1517344999

Cover Picture: Shutterstock

Cover Design: Fiver, by Jeshart

DEDICATION

In loving memory of Michael

And

In Honor of Mark and Charlaine for their undying efforts on his behalf.

Table of Contents

PROLOGUE

"He's gone!"

Those words will haunt me for the rest of my life.

"I came in and tried to wake him; but, he is cold and stiff. Pat, he's gone!"

These were the words of my son, Michael's roommate. Chilling words.

The phone call came at 10:16 PM on Sunday night. The caller was Trey, my son's roommate.

Michael was my oldest son; 48 years old, anticipating his birthday in 3 weeks. Ninety miles away, he lived in a two-bedroom apartment of which he was so proud. Months earlier, he had taken in his friend, Trey, who had fallen on hard times, allowing him to share the place until he found his own. Other friends would come and go as Michael seemed to attract people from all walks of life. He seemed so happy. We had talked on Saturday about his birthday. The future looked bright for him. But now, those dreadful words.

"He's gone!"

How did this happen. Contacting my other children, I paced the floor and recounted his life as a panorama before me.

Chapter One

The Beginning

Michael came to us in February of 1962 when he was six months old. We had been so excited upon learning that a baby boy had been found for us. Having applied to adopt a child a year before, we had been through all of the home evaluations, background investigations, and revealed our finances and physical health reports. Then, we had waited—and waited. When the word finally came that a child had been found, we were beside ourselves.

We were told that this baby had tested with a very high IQ which had led them to place him with us since we were both "educated." My husband had a master's degree and I had some college at that time. But, we were also told that his parents had been "very young"—she was sixteen and the boy was seventeen. They both had been involved with drugs and alcohol quite heavily. This baby had been premature and in the incubator had suffered a seizure which had been attributed to a calcium deficiency. Later, we would learn that he had been born with fetal alcohol syndrome. The mother had wanted to keep him and had moved to our state to live with her grandmother in order to do that. She had also wanted to continue high school and tend to him. However, this became more difficult than she had imagined and after three months she felt unable to cope and had surrendered him for adoption.

Upon being given up for adoption at the age of three months Michael was in five different foster homes in the ensuing three months, we were told. Further, we learned that he had been abused in at least one of them and sexually molested in another. Now, he was to be ours.

When the baby was introduced to us, we were in a hotel room two hundred miles away from our home. The Social Worker presented him in a faded blue blanket wearing worn overalls and socks. We were enthralled! Looking beyond his attire, we saw a fuzz of blonde hair, a complexion so fair that his veins were visible, eyes like a cornflower on a mid-summer day, and an expression that was totally blank. We were told that we could have a trial visit and that the worker would return in three hours to pick him up. With those instructions, she left us alone with him.

With no earthly idea of what to do, we put him on the bed and took off all of his clothes just be sure that he was alright. I still am not sure what we expected. He was amicable to this, however. As directed, we had brought clothing and some toys and bottles. When I redressed him, we gave him the toys--the diversion grabbed his interest.

He looked at first one of us and then the other and the slightest of smiles lit up his face and totally enveloped us. Talking to him, holding him—first one of us and then the other—he responded to both of us; however, he dropped asleep far, far too soon. So, for the remaining time of our visit, we sat and watched him sleep. He stirred occasionally, and made a few baby sounds, but, all in all, it was a quiet moment of perfect serenity and peace.

Sure enough, the worker returned right on time to take him away. This was most traumatic for us. Having waited so long for him and then having him with us, giving him up was a most difficult task. She told us that we would have twenty-four hours to think about him, and if we still wanted him, she would bring him back. She made it very clear that we were under no duress to take him—the decision was to be totally ours

How foolish!

Those minutes spent watching him were precious! There was no way that we would NOT take this child. So, we went to dinner, came back and tried to watch some inane TV program but mostly watching one another and smiling broadly. The decision was made. This was OUR child. Sleep never came to either of us that night. The excitement was too much.

The next morning, when she called, we shared our decision and an hour later she was back with the baby. Again, he was wrapped in the faded blanket and wore the same overalls and socks. The Social Worker directed us to change him into the clothes that we had been told to bring because she would need the ones that he was wearing. She also brought six bottles of formula and asked for the six empty bottles we had been told to bring. The exchanges were made.

We had purchased clothes for the baby as soon as we were accepted. As well, we had outfitted a nursery with a bed, play pen, rocking chair, diapers, clothing, toys, and stuffed animals. Given it a fresh coat of paint and put up some plaques and pictures. The blue corduroy overalls and matching shirt that we had brought along for him fit him perfectly. The little shoes were just right. We had brought two new soft blankets: one was white with thin blue lines forming a square pattern and the other blanket was solid blue. When we returned the clothes, bottles, and blanket, the worker had us sign papers, and then she was gone!

We were alone with our baby!

During the fifth year of our marriage, we had learned that we would be unable to have a child. There was really no discussion: we had always wanted children, so adoption was logical for us. The two long years we had waited allowed us to finish school and move back to our home state, where my husband had been called to his second pastorate. Another year of waiting encompassed the fulfilling of all of the requirements to adopt. Among our many discussions had been the naming of this little boy who would be our son.

First, we considered naming him for our fathers, but that would make his name Freddie Fay. Both of us contemplated his high school years with that name and dismissed it. Several other names were also eliminated before we decided on John Michael—which in Biblical terms means "beloved gift of God." Michael was that to us.

He was the very best baby.

The first night we were a bit apprehensive of how things would go; but, after his bottle, I rocked him to sleep and put him into his brand new bed where he did not utter a sound. He slept all through the night. We were up and down all night to be sure that he was still there and that he was breathing, not because he needed us.

We had a dog, Friskie, who had been with us for five years. Because we were concerned about how she would take to the baby, we had gone to great lengths to introduce her to the baby's room before he came home. Then, we were sure to make a special effort to introduce them when we brought the baby home. She just sniffed and turned away. Imagine our surprise when we went to check on the baby at midnight and there was Friskie asleep under his bed. She did that every night of Michael's life until she died six years later. Even the dog understood that Michael was special to us.

Our families and our church family were aware that we had applied for a baby boy and that we were preparing for him, but the State regulations specified that we could not tell anyone that a child had been placed with us until the visit was complete and we were back at home. We were forbidden from even telling where we had gone to get the child. This was particularly difficult because we had to drive within only a few miles of our parents on the way home with him.

Our church family picked up on the idea that we must have gone to get our child when neither of us were at home for two days and one night without telling anyone where we were going. So, when we drove up to our house, the word spread rather quickly. The telephone calls and visits started within only a few hours. They were all eager to share our happiness.

On the following Sunday, we took Michael to church where he was the center of attention. While Charles preached, Michael slept quietly in my arms, totally unaware of the change he had made in our lives or the lives of those about us.

Shortly, the church family gave Michael a baby shower with all kind of gifts. He slept right through that as well. They gifted us with everything that we could ever have dreamt of having for this little boy. There were little church outfits complete with bow tie, play suits, cloth diapers, toys and everything that one could imagine along with gifts of cash and savings bonds for his college education.

He was such a beautiful baby: so small with blonde hair and blue eyes that missed nothing. One of the most amazing things was that he looked just like my baby pictures. We had been told that the State would do all that they could to match the child to our physical looks and backgrounds. They really did a super job. For the rest of his life, wherever we went, we always heard how much he looked like me. I was thrilled.

During our preparation to adopt, we had promised God that when He allowed us to get a child, we would NOT let that affect our service to the church. We didn't. Michael went to every service of the church. I often joke that he was reared on the back pew of the church. When a nursery was made available, he would stay there where he was so good. If there was no nursery, we would sit on the back pew with a bottle and a few toys. That was the perfect setup until he was about two and a half years old when there was no longer a bottle and he was not sleepy. He would take his little cars and run them up and down the pew, but when he learned to make the "zooooommmm" sound, that was not a good idea. Picture books were good until he wanted me to read to him or talk about the pictures. Not so good either! The worst part of this was that for some reason, he learned to scream. With no warning at all, he would just let out this highly pitched scream. Although it did not last long, it was piercing to the ears of everyone in the church. Many times, I would take him outside so that the service might continue. However, there were times when he was perfect.

Remembering that Michael's IQ had checked out to be high, we were not surprised at how quickly he caught on to the slightest little things. He began to crawl and before we knew it, he was pulling up on anything of substance and then walking. Books were one of his favored toys and he could remember the stories that we would read to him. He began to talk early as well by pointing out animals and learning the sounds they made. He was happiest when we were reading to him. This was about the only time that he was still as well.

Michael gave up on naps very early in his life. He had so much energy and so much to do that he simply could not be bothered with taking time out for a nap. When he was put down for a nap, he would fuss and wiggle. If left alone in his bed, he would play with whatever toy was there for a bit, then stand up and call for someone to come and get him. He tried to climb out of the bed and became successful before we ever would have believed possible. Being still was NOT a part of his behavior. Whatever he was doing had to have action. Bathing him became a chore. He would NOT be still. A simple bath turned into a total dousing of the one attempting to bathe him as well as a soaking for the bathroom.

He loved to play outside in his pool in the summer. One of his favorite times was when I would put him into the stroller and take the dog and walk around the neighborhood. He also enjoyed playing in his room alone with his toys. When he was three, he got a swing set with a slide for his birthday. Did he ever love that! The sand box was a favorite for him and his trucks as well. He amused himself quite nicely. As long as he could be active, he was very happy. We attributed his over activity to just being stubborn and maybe spoiled. We had waited for him so long that we wondered if we were too permissive. Our attempts to control him were tightened and we began to observe carefully his activities only to agree that he was overly active and deliberate.

A small creek ran along the back and side of our yard and Michael knew it was a boundary. He was very good about not playing in the water. Our neighbors across the creek had three stone frogs in their yard. On one of our walks to town, Michael saw and fell in love with them. Imagine how stunned we were to discover that he had crossed the creek and brought the smallest frog to our yard. He tended the frog as if it were alive. Insisting that he take it back, we thought we were being good parents. The next day, we discovered the frog was back in the sandbox again. This became his practice as I patiently explained that the little frog lived under that bush in the neighbor's yard and liked his home. Thinking myself to be so smart, I discovered the frog back within three days. Finally, the neighbors just gave up and gave the frog to Michael. He never forgot that. Each time we moved, the frog went too.

Another neighbor had a garden where he grew a number of vegetables for his kitchen. Among his crops were watermelons. He loved Michael so much that he would pick a watermelon a couple of times a week and roll it down the hill to Michael who loved watermelon. This same man had taken Michael to see his cows and Michael came home determined that he would get a "bull cow." That was all that he talked about for months. Christmas came and Michael asked Santa for a "bull cow." Imagine our surprise when these neighbors gave Michael a ceramic "bull cow" for Christmas. This cow looked just like the cows on the farm.

That same visit introduced Michael to tractors. He wanted a tractor for Christmas as well. This wonderful man took Michael to his farm and would ride with him on the tractor for an hour or so at a time. Imagine how that thrilled this little boy. Everyone at the church knew that Michael wanted a tractor. He told them that "for sure" he was getting a tractor for Christmas. Santa kept his promise and brought a big red metal tractor with pedals that Michael drove for years. That, too, we kept and moved with us. He insisted that it be kept for "your grandchildren." We kept it until Mike was about 45 and we knew that we had all of the grandchildren we would ever have. No wonder Michael felt loved: all of his dreams came true.

Then came a new situation. When Mike was two, we applied to adopt a second son. We made Michael aware that he was going to get a baby brother. We talked about the new child to him and shared the preparations for the new baby. We made a new room for Michael with twin beds and all of his "big boy" toys. He moved his things into the new room and slept there happily as he awaited his little "brudder." The subject of a new little brother was important to him. But, like us, he was anxious to have the baby and get on with the program.

When the new baby was not immediately forthcoming, Mike stopped asking questions and got on with his daily activities. We were equally frustrated but held onto the promise that the new baby would come in time. We tried to keep Mike attuned as the time went on and on. Finally, our patience was rewarded.

Chapter Two

A Brother Comes

When we were preparing Michael for a brother, we shared that the new baby would be named James Mark, which in the Bible means, "a follower of my brother." We were so pleased with our first son that we just knew that another just like him would certainly be a blessing and a joy. Mike had accepted our preparations happily, participating in setting up the nursery and even sharing his stuffed animals in preparation. He had learned to say his nighttime prayers early and began to add a prayer for his brother.

As we prepared for Christmas in Michael's fourth year, we got the word that a second son was available for us. Michael talked about his new "brudder Mark." This waiting interval, we had assumed would be about a year, like Mike. Imagine our lament when it took two years before a child was ready to be placed with us. Remember, we could neither tell Michael that we were going for the baby nor where we were going; so, when we left to get the new baby, as we waited until we were in the car to tell him where we were going. He was so excited!

Unlike the procedure with Michael, the new experience required us to go to the Social Service in another city where we were taken into a room with a mirror that looked into the room where the baby was. There he sat on the floor with a Social Worker playing with a little train. He was nine months old with thin brown hair and the darkest eyes I have ever seen. We lifted Michael up to the mirror and he saw the baby. He clapped his hands and said, “That’s my brudder, Mark!” Insisting that he had to go into that room, the worker had no choice but to introduce him to this new baby. Mike immediately took to the baby and sat on the floor sharing blocks and a ball with him while we watched happily. This unequivocal acceptance and joy continued as we discussed the matter and prepared to take Mark home.

As the Social Services personnel observed the two little boys, they were amazed. At first, Mark drew back and just looked at Michael with those big, dark eyes. But, Mike’s happiness must have been contagious because, when a block was offered to Mark, he took it and that was the beginning of a “play period.”

Normally, we would have taken Mark with us for a few hours to get acquainted; however, because of the obvious ease of relating and because the weather was very cold, the personnel there decided to just let us use that room to become acquainted.

We took turns getting onto the floor with the two boys and playing with them. Mark gave us that serious look and finally a tiny, little smile. He obviously preferred Mike. So, we watched the interplay and reviewed the documents covering Mark’s health and background

When we had to leave, Mike was so disappointed that we were not taking Mark with us. Mark watched the movement seriously, not really sure that what was happening. But, we took Mike and had dinner then back to the hotel where we talked it over—the three of us and decided that Mark was the "brudder" Mike had sought.

The next morning, we urged Mike to dress and have his breakfast so that we could go to get Mark. Of course, there was paperwork before we could even see the baby. We were all anxious, but, the deed was done. After signing the papers—Michael insisted on signing too--we were allowed to take the baby home.

The ride back to our home was interesting. Michael insisted on feeding Mark his bottle. He shared the toys he had brought and wanted Mark to sit in his lap. We were thrilled. Mark went to sleep. Michael had long since given up naps, but he lay beside Mark and was as still as can be. This was amazing!

At home, we rejoiced at the way Michael shared his toys with Mark and included Mark in his activities. Michael would insist on feeding Mark in the high chair and wanted to hold him in his lap often. When Mark awoke at night and cried, Michael was often there by the time I was. Mark became his project. Sitting in church with the two of them was a real experience! Michael quieted down and tended to Mark. The screams stopped because "it scares Mark."

Mark was shy and quiet. At nine months old, he was already sitting alone and tuned in to everything going on about him. His smile was not immediate, but when it came, it was wonderful. Of course, his first smile was to Mike. Mark delayed walking longer than we had anticipated. Through

Mike's efforts, he began to walk. Mike also toilet trained Mark at a VERY early age.

Our life seemed so perfect. We had a lovely home, a marvelous church, and two boys who got along perfectly. As is the case when something seems perfect, the unforeseen intruded into our idyllic lives. Almost overnight there was a dramatic change in Michael's behavior. He was violent, hateful, almost mean refusing to listen to us or to accept our instructions. He threw his toys had terrible dreams that left him screaming. We had no warning and no understanding of what was happening in our home. We were as lost as everyone else. The most notable part of this change was that his protective attitude toward Mark increased. While everything else was falling apart and his behavior was not acceptable at all, he was gentle and kind with our baby, Mark. Not until thirty years later did I know what happened.

When Michael shared the story with his psychiatrist, the doctor insisted that he share it with me. Reluctantly, apologetically he did. Remember now, when he told me the story, he was almost forty years old!

Mark loved his naps. At nine months old, he was always ready for that time of day. Mike would play on his own either in his room or wherever I might be in the house or yard while Mark slept. One day, I was holding a meeting of a church committee at our house while Mark was napping. My neighbor sent her twelve-year-old son over to "entertain" Michael during my meeting. They were busy in his room with a train set, so I went to the living room and my meeting.

Unknown to me for thirty-plus years, the neighbor boy asked Mike to let him see Mark sleeping. There was a bathroom between our room and Mark's nursery, so Mike took the boy through our room into that bathroom so that they could peek at Mark without ever entering his room. Without disturbing Mark's sleep, the boy got his look . . . and more.

The boy urged Mike into the shower and closed the door. There he undressed Mike and fondled his genitals. But, that was not enough, the boy unzipped his pants and compelled Mike to perform oral sex on him. Remember now, Michael was barely four years old and the boy was twelve.

In recounting all of this to a psychiatrist, Mike shared that he thought that they were going to take a shower so he got into the stall and allowed himself to be undressed. When he realized what the boy was doing, he tried to get away but was pushed to his knees and had the penis of the older boy shoved into his mouth. When he tried to get away, he was held in place by the older boy and when he tried to call out, he was threatened.

When the older boy was done, he told Mike that if he ever told about this, Mark would be hurt.

Now, Mark was Mike's new little brother toward whom he felt protective and with whom he had established a good relationship. Apparently, keeping Mark safe was important enough to Mike to never share this information with us. Only as an adult was he able to share and by that time the damage was so far past done that we have only been able to wonder what might have been the difference in Mike's life had we known of this incident. Instead, we allowed this older boy to come into our home on many other occasions to play with and "entertain" both of the boys.

The change in Michael was immediate.

We had no point of reference for why, but things were different. The "change," as we referred to it, was a difference in Mike's attitude and a violent streak in his relationships with others, especially children. He was not as careful with his toys. He acted up in his Sunday school class, in the church nursery, in church, wherever we went. There was an attitude of rebellion in everything he said and did. We were absolutely at a loss to explain how this sunny, smiling little boy became sullen and resenting. Nevertheless, our lives changed from that point on.

Chapter Three

The Change

At this time, Michael was four years old. He had a playmate in a little boy who was five years old who lived around the corner. The two of them had been playmates for a long time. They had shared their toys, spent the night together at his home and at our home. We took the boys with us on outings and thrilled that Michael got along so well with him.

When "the change" occurred, we noticed it first in the way Mike treated this playmate. He fought with him—often biting him on his arms, leaving marks when the boy went home. The mother complained to me. I did not blame her; however, my explanation was inadequate as I did not understand a bit of it either. We kept the boys apart for some time, but when they were together, Mike was vicious to him.

We could tell a difference in Mike's treatment of Mark as well. Perhaps we were seeing Mike's cry for help, but unable to recognize it. One might have construed this change as Mike's resentment of Mark, but that was NOT the case. Mike still showed concern for his brother, but he seemed to want to BE Mark. They shared toys, and eventually a room, and a place in our hearts.

As things worsened, so did Michael's attitude toward Mark. Mike would take things away from Mark. One Christmas, their Aunt Margaret and Uncle Johnny gave each of them a piece of toy construction equipment. Mike's was a bull dozer and Mark's was a road scrape. As they played, Mike took the toy away from Mark by snatching it. Mark burst into tears as Mike began to play with both toys. Margaret immediately made Mike return the toy, admonishing him, "We gave that to MARK—this is yours!" Mike was still determined to have the toy that was Mark's and at the same time unwilling to have Mark play with the bull dozer.

Because Mark was smaller than Mike, this behavior continued for years. Constant vigilance was necessary to assure that Mark had ownership of anything. At the same time, Mike was very protective of Mark when it came to others. He did NOT want Mark to be disciplined at all. When Mark cried, Mike wanted his demands met. These actions were contradictory and we could not understand.

Meanwhile, our work at the church continued. We knew that all of our church family could see that something was wrong. Conferring with our Pediatrician, we were told that this was just a part of his "growing up." Yet, we wondered how that could be. He had been such a sweet little boy and so loving to everyone and now he was "hell on wheels." The people who had indulged him with all kinds of favors were shocked at his behavior, especially the violence.

Everything that Mike did was a full speed ahead. He never walked, he ran. He tumbled down the hills, jumped off of high places, took all kinds of chances. He had no fear!

When he turned five, we enrolled him in Kindergarten. This was supposed to be a time of "socializing" him and getting him ready to go to school the next year. This became a time of increased rebellion against going to school, being at school, coming home from school and after school. We began to see that he resented any kind of authority at all. He indulged us as his parents, but as far as any other rules were concerned he rebelled at them. That meant that school was most disagreeable. Our lives were filled with the stress and tension as well as our fears of what “real school” would bring.

Getting him ready in the mornings was beyond a chore. He did not want to dress, he did not want to get into the car, he did not want to play at home, nothing pleased him. At school, he was uncooperative with the teacher and the other students. He pinched the other children, tried to take the toys they were using and at snack time refused to share but would snatch the snacks of the other children. Continuing complaints from the teacher to us were met with total agreement and we reinforced everything that she recommended. Needless to say, we were beyond embarrassed.

When we went home for Christmas, Mike’s behavior spoiled the happy time for most of the family. He was hateful to his cousins, refusing to play nicely. Efforts on part of his grandparents to placate him by getting him involved in making cookies were met with belligerence and throwing food about the room. Toys did not help. Time outs did not help. Nothing helped. We were glad when we could pack up our children and go home.

After that fiasco, we sought help again but no one could explain what had happened. Mike was uncooperative and really out of control despite our best efforts. Then, our lives took a new turn.

A pulpit committee visited our church and the result was a call to a church in another part of the state. The community was larger, nearer a city where we felt that we could get help for Mike, which we felt might be an answer to our prayers. The church was larger and my husband was a perfect fit to implement and reinforce the programs already in place and institute new ones as well.

Praying for God's will, my husband was led to accept the call to this church which would mean a move of our family and our household to the new church field. By this time, Michael's behavior had gone from bad to worse. The people who had found him so endearing and been a part of his life were more inclined to back off and to join us in wondering what had brought about the change in him. I could not help but wonder if perhaps they were not sorry to see us leave. My father remarked to me when I told him about the move that he had wondered if the church people were not aware that something was really wrong. He, like us, was at a loss to explain. We could only hope that the change of scenery would help us to find the cause and remediate it as soon as possible.

In the ensuing chaos of preparing to move to another church in another town, we convinced ourselves that Michael would be well-served in these new surroundings and forged ahead with the packing and planning. Michael was five years old at this time: Mark was two years old. Neither of them had any idea about what was taking place and just merrily continued with their daily routine of playing and wondering about the plethora of boxes and the sorting of toys and clothing.

One of the first clues that this would NOT be easy came when Michael learned that he could not take his tire swing with him to the new house. When he was about two years old, his Daddy had secured a sturdy rope to an even sturdier tree limb, and attached a car tire to the end making a great swing. Michael instantly fell in love with it and spent hours and hours being pushed out over the yard in that swing. His play pal was terrified of it, but Michael had no fear. Perhaps this should have been a clue that his disposition was making a transition for which we were not prepared. However, when Mark was big enough, he too loved the swing. They even found a way to swing together! Michael enjoyed pushing Mark on the swing and would do so tirelessly. Now, there was no tree at the new place that would hold the swing, so it would be left behind. Not understanding at all, Michael made scene after scene! There was no way to compensate for the loss of the swing. At length, we agreed to take the tire and the rope and try to find a limb. That placated him.

When Mark was a baby, Santa brought a swing set with a slide to the boys together. We assembled the set adjacent to the tire swing and sandbox; but the tire swing had always been the favorite. Even on the day of the move, he would not give up and sat in the swing despite our pleas. When, at length, the rope and tire went onto the van, he had to admit defeat. But, it was not easy.

Many years later, as an adult, Michael went back to that house to see if the limb for his swing was still there. He could not accept that one thing of his could not go with him. We would learn eventually, years later, that this attachment and unwillingness to surrender to others even in the smallest way was a part of the condition that would plague Michael for the rest of his life.

So, we withdrew him from Kindergarten, packed up all of our belongings, our two children and moved.

At any rate, we made the move to our new church field. Confident that the change in location would have a positive effect on Michael and his problems, we set up housekeeping in our new house. As the movers were unloading the van, Michael stood by and when the swing set was brought out, he quickly took over leading them into the backyard and showing them where it should be. He also cajoled some of the men of the church who had come to help set up the furniture and appliances and got them busy setting up the swing set. With Mark by his side, he supervised and when the set was complete, they went right back to playing just as if they realized that this was home. He also saw to it that the precious tire and rope were carefully stored in the shed behind the house for future use. As this unfolded, I prayed that this was a sign that things were going to be better.

Busy with the duties in the new church, Charles was away as the boys and I settled in.

Chapter Four

The Seed Is Sown

Michael had been accepted into a private Kindergarten by virtue of his status as the "Preacher's Son." Alas, our son was not exactly what they were expecting. We learned that despite the fact that he had been in Kindergarten for the entire school year, he refused to do what the other children were doing. He knew his colors, alphabet, numbers, shapes, and the like: he could write his name and could read before he ever BEGAN Kindergarten; he just did not want to participate in activities with the other children. He REFUSED—quite adamantly—to be still much less take a nap at quiet time. This led to unrest among the other children and eventually a mini-revolt! Needless to say, the quiet teacher was NOT happy. We were summoned to conferences and had no explanation for his behavior. Away from the school, we acknowledged to one another that we were no better off in this new location as far as his situation was concerned.

Michael was so energetic that he was almost manic at times. Sleep was very difficult at our house. We would try to "wear him out" with family activities and demanding playtime. Mark would go right to bed at the time set and go right to sleep. Not Mike! He totally rebelled. If forced to go in the room and get into his bed, he would jump up and down, unmake the bed and use the pillows to keep Mark awake. He would throw himself at the walls, bounce on the bed trying to touch the ceiling. He would get out of the bed and empty the toy box to the floor, throw the books from their shelves to the floor, and pull clothes from the closet. Eventually, Mark learned to sleep through it all. But when Mike needed a partner, he would awaken Mark and the crying would ensue. As these episodes became more and more regular, we sought help and moved Mark into the guest room.

The boys had enjoyed separate rooms in our previous home; but, had to share a room now. This was terrible for Mark who liked and needed his sleep. Mark could play quietly and he liked his nap time. Fortunately, Mark had the hours Michael was at school to himself and could play. He would be napping when Mike came home which presented a real challenge. No way in the world would Michael join Mark for a nap; instead, he wanted Mark up to join him in all of the activities he enjoyed.

While Michael was in first grade, the church built a new home for use by their pastor. Almost as an answer to our prayers, the boys could again have separate rooms. When we moved our furniture in, Mark was given the corner room with lots of windows and light as well as a big double bed all for himself. His toys and books were moved in and he set up his room just the way he liked it. Finally, he would have peace separated from Michael with a bathroom that they would share. This reduced the problems of Michael's aggravating Mark as much. In addition, it gave a greater sense of ownership and provided more space for each of them. There were far fewer "fights" at bedtime and greater responsibility for each boy. We thought that this was absolutely wonderful!

Michael was in first grade and having all kinds of trouble in school. His teacher was constantly calling us with reports of his failure to grasp the concepts she was teaching and which the other students were mastering with no problems at all. His behavior was a constant problem. We were summoned to school for conferences and permission to punish Michael for his behavior. Other students complained of his shoving them and trying to fight. He abused all of the materials in the classroom, breaking his own crayons and pencils and trying to take those of other students. In short, it was mayhem.

We knew that he had the IQ to do well in school and were stumped! At home, we would talk to him and talk to him with no connection at all. He hated school. Getting him up in the mornings and to school was a major task. When he came home, he was angry, sullen, and resentful. We prayed for some sort of guidance on what to do. He was miserable and he made all of us miserable.

Increasingly, we were made aware that something was really wrong with Michael. He was maturing physically but emotionally and mentally something was not right. His behavior which had undergone such a great change was deplorable. His proclivity to violence and physical activity was troubling. He continued to bully Mark at home but to be very protective of him when other children were around. He would play nicely with Mark for a time, then without warning lapse into almost punishing him.

We had consulted a new doctor immediately upon moving to this new area, informing him of the first years of Michael's life and the change that had wrought so much havoc for our family. After visiting with Michael alone, he diagnosed him as "simply hyperactive." His recommendation was that we put Michael on medication to "calm" him allowing him to be more attentive in class and control his behavior. After several months of medicating him, we were painfully aware that this was not working. This doctor recommended a Pediatric Psychologist in an attempt to deepen the investigation of Michael's problems.

Fortunately, we were referred to an excellent doctor with these unique qualifications within driving distance of our new home. During an introductory session, we shared what we knew of Michael's background including the seizure in the incubator along with the fact that Michael's biological mother had kept him for three months before surrendering him for adoption which was added into the equation hunting for an answer to Michael's problems. As well, the five foster homes that had followed were considered a factor. One of these homes had resulted in sexual abuse, we had learned, and although he had been removed from that home, this too, was considered a factor. Remember, we knew nothing of the sexual abuse Michael had suffered at age four—three years before—so we could not share this with the doctor. With all of this information, the doctor met Michael and began a series of tests.

After these tests, we learned that Michael was dyslexic—meaning that he saw things from right to left rather than the traditional left to right. While this had not bothered Michael in his reading, there was a major problem with his math skills. To this end, we were informed that special tutoring would be needed. Again, God had led us to this new field of service where we were able to find such tutoring which used the "new found" computer technology to instruct dyslexic students in basic math skills. So, twice a week, I would load the boys into the car and drive forty-five minutes for a one-hour session for Michael.

At first, the newness of the technology appealed to him and he was most cooperative. His grades, however, did not improve and sure enough, when it got old to him, he turned off and refused to cooperate in going to the center or following instructions while he was here. He grew more and more sullen. At length, we were directed to stop the tutoring and bring Michael to the doctor for counseling instead.

During these sessions, the doctor talked with Michael as he endeavored to determine the roots of the problem we were seeing manifested in his everyday behavior. When the doctor met with us, he admitted that there had been little progress. Michael was sullen in his meetings, refusing to talk at all, or only giving one-word answers. This, of course, revealed nothing. So, we were back to square one, dealing with him at home, teaching him how to overcome his dyslexia in math and trying to support his teachers with the behavioral problem

The doctor had led us to examine our own behaviors and how much this might have contributed to Michael's problems. In our sessions, we confessed to the fact that we had waited so long for a child and were so accepting of his initial behavior that perhaps this might be a factor. We had been very careful with Michael from the time he came to us. We watched over him almost to the point of hovering. When he began to walk and manifest his independence, we were very accepting. He had seemed to respond to our loving efforts with smiles, laughs, and love. Indeed, he had blossomed into a physically beautiful and wonderfully loving child. We had taken him everywhere we went and he had responded to people happily. Sure that we had been blessed with perfection and that we were the greatest of parents, we eagerly worked with the doctor to find a solution to what had happened.

Some exploration into the decisions to adopt a second son, and the ways that decision may have affected Michael was made with the help of this doctor. His conclusion was that Michael really loved his brother and that our decision had been perfect because Michael had been eager to share and still had so much consideration for his brother. The doctor told us that Michael could have been damaged further if he had not had someone with whom to share. His conclusion was that Mark had benefited from Michael's efforts to teach him and that Michael had benefited from taking some of that responsibility. His further conclusion was that the bullying Michael was doing to Mark was really an effort to be more like him. To Michael, Mark had no problems: no one was trying to make him do math or control his behavior or attempting to change him in any way. Mark was not being punished, put into time out, or deprived of TV privileges. Of course, Mark was only four years old and had no math to do. Plus, he was a quiet, well-behaved child who was doing nothing to deserve any punishment; however, in Michael's eyes, Mark was his equal. This did seem to be true because the bullying usually came right after Michael was in a tutoring session or being punished for something that he had done.

Totally perplexed and believing that there had to be something that we were missing, we dedicated ourselves to giving the boys the best home life that we could. We taught them to share, to take care of their things, to obey, to be polite and courteous, to say "ma'am" and "sir" and to have proper manners. They said their prayers at night, and blessed their food at each meal. They attended Sunday school and children's church meetings.

Michael played Little League baseball but had MAJOR problems because of his dyslexia. Playing in the outfield, he would move under a ball to catch it; however, he would see it in his brain differently and miss. At the plate, he would be ready to hit, but his brain would misjudge the ball and he would strike out. Trying him a various positions landed him in the outfield. We would watch painfully as fly ball after fly ball eluded him. The coaches and other players were not kind at all. Mike came to the point that he absolutely hated playing baseball. We had purchased a left-hander's glove, but there was more wrong than that. The lack of confidence about the sport led to a resentment of the coach and the team. He came to each game with a chip on his shoulder. Seemingly, no amount of practice helped his game at all. At one game, he missed a ball in right field and the coach punched him. He was six years old. My husband was furious. That night, we made the decision that putting Michael through that was punishment. So, his baseball career ended. Mercifully, the season ended. He never picked up his glove or ball to play with the neighborhood boys or with Mark for the rest of that summer. Instead the sport seemed dead to him.

With Charles increasingly busy at church, I worked with the boys all of the time. We played games, worked puzzles, cleaned house, worked in the yards and just enjoyed being a family. Every effort was made to give both of them a good strong attitude. Sometimes Michael was cooperative and we had a wonderful time. Other times, he was totally the opposite. Mark would try to cope with these mood swings as best he could. My heart went out to him for he had no clue what to expect and too often was the object of Michael's wrath.

Such was our life.

Chapter Five

What Comes Next?

Upon our move, we had decided to adopt another child—this time a little girl. Believing that our ages were fast approaching the upper limit considered positively for adoption, we applied immediately. Michael's adoption had taken a year from our approval for consideration until the child was placed, and Mark's adoption had taken two years. We anticipated at least that long this time. However, to our surprise, our little girl was with us within three months!

Both boys were a bit dubious about having a girl in our house, but as we made the trip to pick her up they got more and more excited over the prospects of a baby. When they saw her, Michael was concerned that she had no hair. For this reason, he did not believe that she was a girl. Having been through this with Mark, he felt like an expert and was advising Mark all along. They were enamored of their little sister, Charlaine. When we told them her name and wrote it out for them, Michael lamented, "She will be in the third grade before she can spell her name!"

Neither boy seemed to mind her being there—there was no obvious jealousy. They delighted in giving her the bottle, putting her to bed, changing her clothes, and trying to get her to talk. She was only three months old, but they wanted action from her. Between the two of them, she was constantly entertained. She walked before she was nine months old—they would not let her crawl at all. She was talking in sentences very early in order to converse with then. There was no baby talk—they wanted "real talk."

Michael's behavior around her was wonderful. He treated her like a baby and a little girl directing Mark to do the same. For the rest of his life, Michael was so very close to Charlaine. He was her protector and she was his buddy. He taught her all about football and she was always ready to play with him when Mark was tired. The union between the three of them was perfect. The idea that these three would never have even met in life had they not come into our home was breathtaking. They were truly siblings. This was a wonderful thing to behold.

While all of this was going on, Michael did progress through the second grade. He made some friends with boys at school as well as boys from the church and in the neighborhood. Being the "Preacher's Kid" was a real burden for him. No matter where he was, people were watching him—and, unfortunately, he was not discreet in his behavior. Seemingly, the older he got, the more antagonistic he became. He wanted to listen to no one. Authority of any kind presented a problem for him. Thus, he had major problems at school, at church, and at home. He picked fights—literal fights—with the neighbor boys. He refused to obey his teachers and just turned off on school. Despite our best efforts to understand and to amend the situation, we were failing.

He had severe problems in his third grade year. The teacher was older and very experienced. She taught in a straight-forward, nuts and bolts style which demanded specific student behavior. The emphasis on “understanding” the individual student, learning styles, and adapting teacher methods was not her style. She expected proper student behavior which meant attentive attitude, participation only when called upon, and respect. Students LEARNED in her classroom which meant that she promoted students prepared with the basics of education—a firm foundation upon which future teachers could build. Many years later, I would come to understand and appreciate this teacher when I had my own students.

Needless to say, Michael was totally at sea in this teacher’s class. He could not, or would not, sit still. Nor, would he keep quiet. She gave a goodly amount of homework with which we labored nightly. He was disciplined severely and regularly: he stayed after school almost daily which was her way of punishment. We were summoned to the school where we listened to lengthy diatribes about his lack of discipline, refusal to participate in classroom activities, lack of attention, and inability to learn. As a direct result of these conferences, we sought additional help for him.

Because the doctor with whom we had consulted earlier had attributed his problems to hyperactivity, we began drug therapy designed to alleviate these problems. While this had not been successful previously, we agreed to try it again. This made him very drowsy and contributed to inattention problems. At this time, we sought a more focused tool to help him.

Having searched for help with his academic problems, we turned again to the individualized tutoring to augment classroom learning using computer technology. There was no interaction with other students nor with a teacher which removed the authority figure problem as well as the social component. Because he was left-handed, his teacher had decided to make him right-handed. Utilizing the computer technology eliminated that particular problem since there was no preference for right or left hand.

Evaluation had indicated that his only real learning problem with Mathematics. So, we made the decision to focus on math only with high hopes for the desire outcome. Much to our disappointment, this activity did not help him at all. At first he was intrigued by the interaction with the computer and the opportunity to work alone. There was instant improvement in his attitude and in his school work. However, after only a few weeks, the newness wore off again. He was sullen during the trips to the Center and uncooperative in the program. His great start was soon diminished by his refusal to continue with the program although we kept at it for the entire school year. Obviously, there were some positive results because he was passed to the fourth grade with satisfactory marks in every subject but with a note of caution regarding his behavior in the classroom, with other students, with the teacher and a total disregard for learning in general.

By the next school year, the schools in our county were integrated by federal mandate. This totally changed the learning game plan for our school which actually benefitted Michael. New and younger teachers were brought in and with them came a different style of classroom management and presentation: new and up-to-date textbooks and resource materials captured his attention as well as associating with new students. At last, we seemed to have a ray of hope. This lasted for three school years and gave us breathing room at home. He still was restless and resentful of authority; but, he was more cooperative. His grades did show some improvements in all areas.

At home, there was a greater sense of peace. Mark had started school by this time and Michael seemed to realize that school was not a punishment being exacted on him alone. He seemed to think that if Mark was going too, perhaps it might not be so bad. Mark had no trouble with learning and his teachers reported only good things about his interaction with others and his general classroom behavior. What a relief that was! Michael seemed to take note of that as well.

About this time, Michael found sports—baseball had not been good for him, but he found football.

During our sessions with the psychiatrist, we had shared the baseball problems. As he explained the difficulties Mike endured as a result of his dyslexia, he stressed the strong need to help Michael to find an activity in which he could engage and find a sense of accomplishment and security despite this handicap. We realized that this was a part of Mike's envy of Mark who was confident in his own skin and eager to be a part of any activity and made friends easily.

Because his father had played football and loved the sport, he keyed in on Mike's love for rough activities, we bought him a football and put him into that program. He loved it! The team spirit seemed good for him and he loved the running and constant physical activity. He wanted to learn to kick so that he could enter the Punt-Pass-and-Kick Contest. He worked endlessly setting up the tee and kicking. Mark and Charlaine were so patient in running to get the ball and bringing it back so that Michael could kick again. This went on for days and days and days. Sure enough, when the competition came, Michael had the confidence not only to show up but to take his turn. All of us shared his joy when he placed third and got a small trophy. We were onto something.

When Michael began to make some efforts toward getting along with his peers, we were overjoyed. Since football only lasted a few months, we had to augment it with something else. Scouting became an outlet for him. He loved being outside and using that as a learning laboratory suited him perfectly. The program was ideal for him and he took to it immediately. At this time, he also went to Royal Ambassador Camp with our church group. The camping lifestyle fit him perfectly. Trapping, fishing, tracking—every facet of the life suited him. That Christmas he received his heartfelt wish—Santa brought him a .410 rifle, a tent, and a sleeping bag. He had his scouting knife, mess kit, snake bite kit and fishing equipment. Plus, he had the desire to put it all together. He and Mark put the tent up in the backyard as soon as weather permitted. Although Mike was far more excited about all of this than Mark, the younger brother went along with it. By this time, the brotherhood between the two of them had begun to manifest itself quite positively. They went to Royal Ambassador Camp together, but were in separate groups. Mark would go on to become a Counselor at this camp and a summer employee during his senior year in high school and all through college. The outdoor life that occurred here took root and lasted for the rest of the life of both boys.

During this time, both boys made a profession of faith in Christ and were baptized joining the church. Because their father was their pastor, he would baptize them. At first, Michael was very concerned that his father would drop him in the pool or might hold him under the water too long. Mark was not concerned at all. On the night of their baptism, he brought both boys into the pool at the same time which made for a moving experience in our church. Amazingly, no one was dropped and the baptism went off without a catch. For the rest of his life, Michael would share that experience insisting that "something happened to me in that pool, I know it did." This became his mantra for showing that he was a Christian and that he was God's child.

While there was real progress for Michael after the diagnosis of his dyslexia, he still struggled with behavioral issues. He was aggressive with his friends to the point of actual physical fighting. One boy in our neighborhood about Michael's age was just as aggressive and they came to blows several times. Neither the boy's mother nor I could blame the other child for we knew it was mutual. We forbade Michael from playing with that boy, but they still found ways to get together and fight. Other boys were his friends and they played ball and camped together, but Michael was always on the edge, almost daring someone to cross him. One would think that Mark would follow him into this, but Mark remained passive and had his own set of friends. Mike seemed to believe that he was different from Mark. He saw Mark as a person whom everyone realized was wonderful, and which meant that there was something wrong with him. He simply could not accept that basing his life on the approval of others or trying to be Mark was a big mistake.

One of the factors that bothered us so much was Michael blaming things on Mark. Because Mark was so quiet and obedient, we could usually tell when Michael was lying. One time, we discovered the back of the television had been taken off while the set was playing. Upon inquiry, Michael "admitted" that the picture had gotten "blurry" and Mark had taken the back off and "fixed it." Immediately, visions of electrocution came to our minds. Their father took a belt and whipped Mark VERY severely. All of the time, Mark was crying and insisting that he had not touched the TV. He never said that Michael did it, but he cried and cried throughout the worst whipping of his life. Because we knew that Michael was capable of lying, he was whipped too. Of course, he too cried and cried protesting his innocence.

Years later, Michael would confess that he, not Mark, took the back off. To this day, I regret that incident. Michael apologized to Mark many times in his later life for "being so mean" to him. Mark's good heart and love for his brother never turned on Michael, but took the abuse, the teasing, and the punishment. When Michael was in the last years of his life, he told Mark, "Take $1,000.00 out of my checking account because I was so mean to you." Mark never did.

Michael was in the sixth grade when we again changed churches and moved to a new town, new house, and a new chapter in the life of our family.

Chapter Six

Trying to Cope

Moving to a new town can be physically demanding for a family. Settling into a new home calls for real effort—physically, mentally, and emotionally. Where the boys had enjoyed their separate rooms with their own bathroom, they now shared a room and shared a hall bath with Charlaine. The entire family experienced the change from a large, brand new home to a much smaller and older home.

As a result, there was less room for our family members to call their own. The church was a driveway's width from our house and the high school was less than a block from our front door. The elementary school was a mile away. The community was very small with very little commerce and a small shirt factory. The idea of fading into the background definitely would not work here.

We did have a large back yard with an old garage at the back. We added a basketball goal and a trampoline for the children. Our goal was to give the children a sense of ownership in this new location. Immediately, Michael decided that the old garage would become their "headquarters."

The physical closeness required all of us to sacrifice some of the privacy and separation to which we had become happily accustomed. This was especially true for Michael. He needed room for his physical pursuits. Mark was given to less physical pursuits and settled right in. Where Mark liked to spend time alone doing homework, he now had to deal with Michael's active presence. Their room lay between the kitchen and the hall, so the lack of privacy was very real. Michael assumed that all of the house was free run for him. No room was off limits at any time, nor were any possessions.

This created problems for Charlaine—as a little girl, she wanted and deserved privacy. Even though she was young, she tried to convince Michael that when her bedroom door or the bathroom door was closed, that meant "KEEP OUT!" Our efforts to demand respect for her privacy and Mark's things met with a deaf ear and dismissal. He did not like the new place and did not care about anyone or anything else.

So, while all of the rest of us adjusted to the new environment, Michael just simply could not or would not. A new school, new house, new church, and new geography presented challenges at every turn for him. With so much grief, we realized that most likely all of the progress he had made as far as interacting and trying harder in school might likely be negated. We prepared ourselves to try to find ways to motivate him again. How could we do all of this all over again?

School was perhaps the greatest problem. Because he had not been a good student—either academically or behaviorally—in his last school, the first day did not reflect our hopes and our efforts. Not surprisingly, he liked neither his new teachers nor the school itself. He felt that the teacher was picking on him because he was new: the "other kids" were "looking at him"; the books were different; the rules were "crazy."

Of course, as his mother and experienced with his school problems, I had high hopes that the change in learning environments would somehow appeal to Michael, and I refused to have my thoughts diminished by the dismal first day. Michael took his frustrating experiences out on Mark and Charlaine by pushing, shoving and hitting them. He kept changing the channels on the TV set to keep them from watching their favorite show. When one of them picked up a toy or a book, he snatched it: when Charlaine went to the slide, he pushed her away: when Mark got on the trampoline, Michael pushed him down and finally off. He refused to behave at the dinner table and argued with his father about the positive points of this new place. Getting him to take his bath and get ready for bed was a battle royal. Long after the lights were out, he was up playing with toys, emptying the closet and awaking Mark.

And this was just the first day!

The next afternoon, the neighbor children came to our house attracted by the basketball goal, swings, trampoline, and the curious "new people." Within the first hour, Michael was in a fight with the boy next door and had two little girls crying. We had rules for playing with others, of course, but Michael totally ignored them. He took the bike from one little boy and rode away despite being summoned to return.

That day was a disaster too!

Recalling the doctor's finding that Michael had problems with authority, we tried to explain anew to him that not only was adjusting to school and the "newness" absolutely necessary, but getting along with his peers was vital. He was unwilling to make any compromise. We agonized over the disrespect he showed for his teacher: the relationship—or the lack of it—with his peers was bad enough but his treatment of adults became increasingly indifferent and aggressive.

Church was equally problematic. He refused to sit still during worship or to take part in children's activities. In the children's choir, he would stand with them but that was as far as he would go. He would pout and distract others. All of the children complained about his kicking and pinching. Sitting with him in church services, I would try to entertain him with books to keep him still and preclude his making a scene. Many times I resorted to removing him from the sanctuary and punishing him for his behavior. This was uncomfortable for both of us and, I admit, accomplished nothing. He was no happier or calm in the new location than he had been in the old. He may have been worse.

We adopted a strict schedule for the children: Charlaine who was now four years old would be relegated to her room during the time that Michael and Mark did their homework. She would not practice piano nor watch TV. One of the boys would work at the dining room table and the other would work at the kitchen table—there was no room in this house for desks for them. If one of them had no homework or finished early, he would go to their room and play quietly or read until the other was done. There would be no TV on in the house during homework time. This helped for a while. Michael's grades actually improved. Both this respite was short lived.

When we were summoned to school for his lack of progress and his misbehavior, we felt stymied. After hearing all of his antics and because we were aware of the problems at home, we decided to consult the professionals again. The school personnel, including the teachers and counselors were eager to hear our story and promised their cooperation. So, we found another psychologist fifty miles away who dealt with adolescents. All of Michael's files were forwarded to him. When we sat down with him to review the files and add our own input regarding Michael's daily behavior and attitude along with the school's findings, the doctor was eager to meet with Michael.

Remember again, at this time, we were unaware of the sexual assault when Michael was four years old; therefore, we could not make the doctor aware of that mitigating factor.

Michael began to see the doctor weekly. Following several visits and extensive testing, the doctor diagnosed him as ADHD (Attention Deficit Hyperactive Disorder) and prescribed a drug to help deal with this disorder. We were advised that with the regular dosage of the medication, we should see a positive change in Michael that would become progressively more pronounced. Needless to say, we were encouraged.

Upon sharing this finding with Michael's teachers, we found all of them to be most cooperative. They really had Michael's welfare prominent in their concerns.

At first, Michael was agreeable to seeing the doctor and taking the medication. He seemed to really make a genuine effort to cooperate with the plan. Our reports from the previous doctors were honest in reporting him as cooperative and open part of the time, and sullen and unresponsive at other times. The report emphasized that many times he would pout and refuse to talk at all. We were the eternal optimists. We had high hopes. You see, we could remember the bright, happy, smiling little boy who had endeared himself not only to us but to the entire community and church family. We remembered how much he loved books and was so eager to read. We also remembered how loving and kind he had been and how proud we had been of him and the sunny disposition and outgoing attitude. We wanted that back. Yes, we had high hopes.

Because I was the one driving Michael to these weekly appointments, I was well aware of the almost violent shifts in behavior. He would often be belligerent and even try to get out of the car while we were driving along. On the occasions that I brought Mark and Charlaine along, he would pick fights with them, hitting and punching them in the back seat. On the days we were alone, he would often play the radio and be content for the trip. Other times he might be totally uncommunicative. The worst were the time he would pout and be verbally abusive during the drive. He would spout vitriol about the place we lived, the house, the church, his things, and his entire world. However, there were times when he was actually enjoyable! Always the trip back home was quiet.

One of the most disturbing factors at this time was his appearance. His complexion became sallow, beneath his eyes, he was almost black, like a bruise. He kept his head down and when he did look up, he had a pouty look with his teeth clenched and his lips tightly drawn. At times his eyes blazed with aggression and antagonism; but, most disturbing were the times when his eyes were flat with absolutely no emotion or feeling at all. To me, this was terrifying.

Even though we kept to our family schedule, Michael's grades fluctuated. His actions within the family were still aggressive. He was often moody and unkind to others. His major victim, unfortunately, was Mark who was longsuffering. Michael's relationship with his peers was not good. He was quick to fight: always on the defensive. I think that the phrase is, "He had a chip on his shoulder." The problem was that he seemed to beg for someone to knock it off. He bullied his siblings and friends alike. Real fights were not unusual.

The redemption of the time was Boy Scouts. Michael anticipated these meetings with a positive attitude. He loved the concept of scouting and embraced the philosophy. The goal he set for himself was to become an Eagle Scout like his idol, Alan Shepard. He worked tirelessly toward that goal. Had he given that much attention to his school work, what a joy that would have been! But, realizing that he had found something about which he felt passionate was certainly positive. While getting him to dress up for church was a real effort, he was eager to get into his scout uniform with all of the patches. He was not aggressive at scout meetings which was another positive. We committed to scouting and helping him attain his goal in any way possible, including letting him make decisions to encourage self-confidence and responsibility. The situation was most encouraging.

Because scouting included camping, Michael really felt that he had found his niche. He went to Boy Scout camp in the summers and came home excited and fulfilled. He was earning badges for doing the things he really loved. We saw a real change in him.

But, then, school began and we were back to square one. Where he had enjoyed the outdoors at camp, school was confining; the activities of school did not compare to the hunting, fishing, and camping. To make matters worse, the penchant Michael had for choosing friends who did not bring out the best in him reared its head again. The boys with whom he chose to hang out were older than he, were repeating the grade because of previous failure, and into marijuana significantly. Because of my husband's position in the community, insisting that Michael NOT associate with these boys became more and more difficult.

With an emphasis on Boy Scouts, we were able to refocus Michael onto a path that incorporated school, church, and leisure time into one activity goal. This left little time to associate with the questionable boys except at school. This seemed to be working along with keeping him on the hyper meds and seeing the psychologist regularly.

In the midst of our search for answers and a workable plan that would provide Michael with a normal, happy life and dealing with his unpredictable actions, we moved again.

Chapter Seven

Very Good and Very Bad

Our new church was in North Georgia and actually nearer our families than we had even lived since our marriage. To Michael's eyes, this new location was a good move. The church, while larger, was not "in town" but in the more rural suburbs where homes were not close together. Indeed, the home furnished for the pastor here sat across the highway and up a hill from the actual church building and was surrounded by woods. Quickly, he inventoried the area by hiking through the woods and finding a neighborhood about a mile or so into the hike through the dense pine forest. Our yard was spacious with plenty of room for the basketball goal, trampoline, and swing set. The children were all pleased. Of course, we experienced relief at Michael's reaction.

The boys again shared a room, but it was quite large with plenty of closet space and space for each of them to personalize to their own interests. Charlaine's room was across the hall, but she shared a hall bathroom with the boys. Because Michael still disrespected the privacy of both Mark and Charlaine, we realized that we had a real problem. With no lock on the door of the hall bath, Charlaine especially was at his mercy. Since the Master Bathroom opened onto the hall as well, we gave Charlaine the use of it to spare her Michael's intrusions. This worked, fortunately. Ironically, being able to have his things separated from Mark's seemed to please him. He put his gun rack over his bed with both of his guns there and his books beside his bed. We were so happy that we actually began to relax.

The church was even pleasant for him. There was an active group of boys and girls his age. By this time, Michael was thirteen years old, so being a part of a group would have been expected; however, he preferred the role of loner. But, for about a year, his reactions to others and the aggression seemed to abate. He made friends with two boys who lived nearby and were well-behaved. Living with their grandparents, they were disciplined and all of their activities monitored. This was a good relationship which we fostered. Michael seemed to enjoy most of the church activities. He was not well-behaved most of the time; but the obvious irreverence was more or less contained. He sat with his peers in worship and seemed to mirror their respect. Again, we were pleased and began to take deep breaths again.

Michael attended the county high school which was enormous. Charlaine and Mark attended the nearby Elementary school. All three of them had to ride a bus to school—well they rode different buses since they went to different schools but they were all subjected to bus transportation. Unfortunately, this proved to be fatal for Michael's problems. The presence of older students—especially boys—had interesting effects on Michael. He selected role models from boys who were not what we would have chosen. Their activities prompted Michael to emulate them and even return to the impossible behavior we had worked so hard to overcome. Added to the problem were the new experiences of smoking, profanity, and disrespecting girls. Riding the bus with these boys gave Michael a new dimension for his difficult behavior.

Since he was now in high school, we tried to impress upon him the importance of good grades for his future—college, career, etc. Unfortunately, this admonition dealt with issues he did not consider "cool." He was intelligent enough to be able to pass all of his classes without giving himself over to studying and homework. He was in class every day and—fortunately—most of the material seemed to stay with him in order to earn passing grades. However, his attitude in class was resentful and reflected total disinterest. He was old enough to realize that his poor behavior of the past was childish so his teachers reported no problems in that regard. But, he continued to be a problem on the bus.

One evening, I got a phone call from a mother of one of the girls on Michael's bus. She related to me how Michael had harassed her daughter for some time with the last episode going over the top. The girl was quite attractive and very smart. Why Michael selected her to annoy, I will never understand. Michael had been teasing her on this day and she was irritated enough to respond angrily to him whereupon he looked around the bus and realized that his little cabal of "friends" were watching and he made a revolting remark about the girl. Of course, she had come home weeping. The remark was so disparaging that I was offended myself! When we confronted him, he denied that it had happened and that he had no knowledge of it whatsoever. After speaking with me, the mother reported the incident to the school and Michael was suspended. Until his death, he continued to deny that he had made the remark, but he paid the price for it with the school and with us.

This was not Michael's first suspension.

Upon our move, I had begun to work now that Charlaine was starting to school. Fortunately, I had gotten a position as a Teacher's Aide in the Elementary School where both Charlaine and Mark were students. For this reason, I was doubly concerned when we got a call from the high school summoning us for a conference. At that time, we were told that the entire school had been in an assembly in the gym—the purpose was to observe Black History day. As it turned out, Michael and one of the boys from the school bus were discovered crawling along the narrow steel girders in the small space along the beams of the roof above the floor the gym itself. We were told in emphatic terms of the danger to which Michael had exposed himself and those beneath him in addition to his skipping the assembly itself. He was suspended for three days. Of course, he denied that he had been in danger at any time, much less exposed others to danger. His suspension delighted him! We were appalled.

Of course, this little event led to punishment at home as well as the punishment from the school. Each morning when I left for school, I gifted him with a list of tasks to be performed that day. Among those tasks were doing the laundry, raking leaves in the yard, cleaning the bathroom, doing the dishes, vacuuming, reading the assignments from school and completing them to our satisfaction and any other incidentals that crossed my mind. Because his father's study was at the church he was nearby to pop in to see how things were going and to come home for lunch and check on the progress. Despite his complaining and arguing about it, he was made aware that there was a penalty to pay when one disobeyed the rules. Needless to say, he was not happy on his "vacation" from school.

Michael's affection for scouting had carried over with this move. Scouting had captured his imagination and interest to the point that he inquired about the possibility of continuing his membership in this new location. We found a local troop which he eagerly joined. The group was quite active with a caring Scoutmaster. The achievements of scouting with its badges and ranks gave him the opportunity to explore a variety of experiences and he threw himself into it. His sash became filled with badges for his many achievements from cooking to knot tying to Morse Code and on and on. His crowning achievement was the night he became an Eagle Scout. He had earned the God and Country award, an honor he cherished, but the Eagle had been his goal and his pride in achieving it was evident. He went on to earn five palms to add to his Eagle.

For us, the experience was more than a ray of hope for Michael and his problems. We saw his embracing of the Code of Scouting as an important step toward overcoming some of the problems with self-esteem and confidence. Then he went to Boy Scout Camp. . .

This was to be an outdoor camping experience which he anticipated with great joy. Assuming a positive outcome, we were stunned when he came home and revealed a black cross tattoo on his bicep. In explanation, we learned that the older boys had forced him to submit and tattooed him with needles and black India ink in the shape of a rough cross. Assuring us that it was all against his will, we pursued the matter with the Scoutmaster and BSA to no avail; but we did take him to a plastic surgeon and have it removed. That was a painful experience for him from which he took away even more anger and loss of self-esteem. Whether or not he was telling us the truth, we never knew. The other boys told the Scoutmaster that Michael had wanted the tattoo and they had only done it with his permission. So, we never knew for sure. One thing we did know, for his entire life, he valued his Eagle Scout experience, the skills he learned in scouting and the love and respect for the outdoors.

Another of the great experiences in this location was Michael's love for the woods and outdoor experiences. With Mark and/or some other friends, he would spend hours roaming the woods near out home. Our boys had the tent and sleeping bags they had gotten for Christmas and put them to great use. They spent every weekend in the woods. Even as an adult, he claimed this period as his happiest memory of his youth and living in this location as his favorite of all the places he lived.

Not an outstanding scholar, Michael was "lost" in the large consolidated county high school. He felt no loyalty or school spirit at all. Football was a passion for him. We always felt that it was a way to expend his aggression and an allowable outlet for the bundled emotions that bugged him constantly. His ability to focus on a limited objective made him shine. Since he would not try out for the school teams, we enrolled him in a county program where teams were fielded by age and geographic location. He was "drafted" by the Cowboys and quickly proved himself as a defensive lineman. The coach of the team was thrilled with his performance and made him a starter. All of us were so proud of him and he knew that he had found his niche. As we attended the games, we could literally see his development and the confidence that it bred. When he was presented with a trophy for outstanding play at the end of the season, his grin revealed a side of him we had never seen.

Coupled with his Boy Scout Eagle award experiences, this was Michael's apogee. Having gotten his driver's permit, we were guardedly optimistic that things were looking up.

Trying to stay abreast of what was going on with him, we saw contradictions in his life. Where he excelled in Scouting and the learning it required, he was willing to bomb in school and stayed on grade level with a minimum of effort: where he excelled at football with the discipline for long and repeated practices, he failed miserably with his personal behavior and attention to social parameters.

Unfortunately, we had no access to a professional to help us to understand and cope. The doctor with whom we had been working upon our move to this location moved away and left us with suggestions which we put with those of the doctor with whom he had been working formerly. At the same time, we were struggling with the fallout of Michael's attitude and actions with his siblings. We were compelled to expend so much time, energy and concern on the problems of one child that I feared that the other two were too often ignored or neglected.

Mark—three years younger than Michael—was also in Scouting where his interest waned until he no longer went to meetings nor worked on his badges. He did participate in the "camping out" but he was never as motivated in that area as Michael. Mark was an excellent student and proved himself a leader despite the fallout from Michael. In his elementary school, Mark was very popular with both the faculty and his peers. His personality was not forceful, but friendly and sincere. He played football in the same county program as Michael and was well-liked. When he went into Middle School, his positive outlook and low-key personality assured him of continuing popularity with both boys and girls as well as the faculty and staff. Involved in extra-curricular activities, he seemed to compartmentalize the problems with Michael and make his own way. Often the victim of bullying from Mike, he maintained a brotherly allegiance and tried—with mixed results—to overlook the situation.

Michael would taunt him and call him names, often in front of his friends. Because of the difference in ages, Michael was bigger which made the bullying ever more difficult for Mark. They had few friends in common—Michael's were louder and prone to trouble with academics while Mark's were more polite and low key as well as academic. The difference in the two boys was noticeable to all.

On the other hand, Charlaine—seven years younger than Michael—seemed quite oblivious to all that was going on around her. She would often try to intervene in the spats between the two boys. Her interest was in music where she would "lose" herself at the piano. A good student, she was placed in the accelerated program during first grade and she continued to excel. With an outgoing personality, she became a cheerleader in the county athletic program where both boys played football. She was placed on the same team as Mark which led to a new relationship between the two of them.

She did become the target of much abuse from Michael on two fronts. He continually bullied her about her weight—she had not lost her baby fat and was a bit chubby—and to tease her about being a girl—over which she had no control whatsoever. But, to the consternation of everyone, an unholy allegiance developed between Michael and Charlaine. She had absolutely no interest in the camping activities, but would visit them at their camp site before dark and run their errands.

When he was not making her cry, she was his chief defender and he would enlist her in many of his activities. The two of them would team up to prank Mark, much to his consternation. This special relationship would last throughout Michael's lifetime. On the night of his death, when she got the news, her husband told us that she almost passed out. Her grief knew no bounds. When she arrived by plane, her tears were still falling, her face was puffed with grief, and she was totally spent. The two of them were that close.

As all of this was unfolding in our home, there was tension between us as parents. Charles was not very understanding of Michael and continued to look upon all of his problems as plain misbehavior which could be ameliorated by using a belt to punish him. As well, he saw the bullying of Mark by Michael as an indication of weakness on Mark's part and refused to intervene. He was very proud of Michael's football achievements, attending every game and encouraging him to "hit harder" and to "be tough." We could all hear him calling out during the game for Michael to "hit somebody" or "go for that number 12." This encouraged Michael to be even rougher and almost violent at times. All told, the appearance was often approval of Michael with pride in him or disapproval with punishment. He was sure that Michael would "outgrow it."

I, on the other hand, felt that the basic problem we had been working on for ten years was being manifest in the varying moods exhibited by Michael and penchant to hurt or abuse others. I tried to talk to Michael and point out the problems, the adverse attitude, the need for focus on his actions, behavior and life in general. Always, I was met with respectful listening and positive responses with promises of change.

But nothing changed. He was out of control and totally anti-social.

With our lives as a family in total turmoil, we received the news that we were moving again. This caused major upheaval among our family members beginning with Michael. He did NOT want to give up his friends—even though most of them we found unsatisfactory—and the woods where he camped. Mark was blindsided and unhappy with the idea of leaving the school where he excelled and the church where he was popular and happy. Charlaine, not a third-grader, was the least upset. None of us could have imagined the impact of this move.

Chapter Eight

Things Go Awry

Just the rudiments of making this move to a new church field almost two-hundred miles away became harrowing. The new house was large enough for each child to have a separate bedroom. As well, there was a large family room in addition to a formal living room. This was a real plus for Mark because he would have his sanctuary. Again, however, the three of them would have to share a hall bathroom.

Because we lived so near the county line, our children would attend school in the nearest town although it was a different county. That meant riding the bus again for all three of them. The high school which Michael would attend was much smaller even though it too was a county high school. We believed that this would be a real plus for him. Mark would have one more year in the middle school and Charlaine would be in the elementary school—all three were separate buildings in different parts of the town.

The yard of our home was large enough for a pool. While the home we were leaving was in the county about eight miles from a town with no close neighbors, the new home was within a small town with close neighbors. The children would be able to walk to town and ride their bikes anywhere that they wanted to go. In our minds, we saw this as an excellent situation for the three of them.

When assessing the overall effects of the move, we felt a tiny positive sense of betterment for Michael. The wisdom of that assessment remained to be seen. We did feel that the pieces were all there to create success if we could just keep them in place appropriately.

In order to physically make the move, we had to determine how to move three vehicles—my car, my husband's car, and a small van we had used in the mission ministry of the church. The church had given us the van as part of our parting gift. After much discussion, the decision was made to have Michael drive the van although he had only a learner's license. Mark would ride with him and they would carry the mattresses so that we could spend the night in our new home while we awaited the moving van with all of our possessions. We could form a motorcade—Charles would lead us; Michael would follow him and I would bring up the rear in my car with Charlaine riding with me.

This decision energized Michael. The fact that we had that much confidence in him seemed to really impress him. Suddenly, he was acting more in control and accepting of the move. In short, he was delighted.

The move was accomplished with a degree of ease that we could never have imagined. We began to look toward to establishing a life in this new location. First order of business was to get the children enrolled in school. The excellent reputation of the system had been a mitigating factor in our decision to cross the county line. This would prove to be a wise decision on our part.

Because the system was so much smaller than the former one, transferring was not a problem until we got Michael to the high school. In an effort to follow his former courses as closely as possible, the school found a way to set him up exactly. However, this, we soon realized, was not to Michael's liking: he balked at resuming ANY math at all. As a mid-term sophomore, this was required. The strength of his rebellion was such that the Counselor agreed to put him into a low-level math class, assuring him that he would have success there. At length, he calmed down, but declared that he would NOT pass the class. By that time, the Counselor had lost patience since no amount of reasoning or threatening or cajoling was helping at all. Deeply within my soul, I felt a little voice warning me of "trouble ahead." There were ten weeks left in the school year and already he was disillusioned.

As a firm believer in sunshine following the rain, we were thrilled when Michael's attitude really began to improve. His classes were NOT the reason—nor his friends. The reason was FOOTBALL.

Michael approached us with the idea of "going out for" the high school football team. After he had enjoyed the experience in our previous location with the community league team, he wanted to "give it a shot." Of course, we encouraged him! Seeing him elect to do something knowing the requirements for participation and maintaining his grades would be necessary, we were thriledl. He insisted that he was ready for it. And, we heartily endorsed the decision. Immediately, we saw an improvement in his attitude, behavior, grades, and family relationships. We were euphoric and totally cooperative!

Football practice began and he measured up—he was very tired at the end of each day, but it was a good tired. The coach elected to make him a starter in the Spring Scrimmage game. Michael was thrilled. We sat in the stands beyond excited at the display of team work, sportsmanship, and attitude. He was good! He seemingly had found his spot and committed himself.

School ended and Michael and Mark spent their summer working in the tobacco fields of South Georgia from sunup to sundown. At first, the sheer labor took a toll on Mike's body, but he accepted the challenge. Shortly, he had become accustomed to the task and the knowledge that he was building up his body for football gave him additional incentive.

At the end of the summer, he was up and at school for practice at sunrise then back to the fields, home for a shower and back to football practice as the sun set. He was home at eight or so for dinner and early to bed. None of us could believe that he would keep this rigorous schedule, but he did.

With the new school year, we lived holding our collective breath to see what would happen as he began his junior year as a member of the varsity football team—a starter at that. We were overjoyed with his reaction to the grade requirements and that the Coach, to whom Michael responded positively, provided tutoring for any player with academic problems. Michael attended these sessions and as a result passed his first math class!

On the football field, he was a dynamo. The number of tackles and assists was impressive and the team and coaches totally embraced him. This experience was brand-new to him and he thrived!

When the season ended and winter set in, he had the serious mood swings, depression and antagonistic traits returning. We were desperate for something that would interest him to keep him involved. Praying fervently that God would see our need and help us find a way to meet it. Our prayers were answered.

One of our church members had a rather large farm out in the country between our little town and the town where Michael went to school. Michael had done part of his tobacco work with him the past summer and apparently had impressed him. Shortly after the new year began, he offered Michael a job after school every day driving a tractor and helping to clear the fields for the new planting season. With an eagerness that surprised us all again, Michael accepted the job offer.

We sat down with him and came up with a plan that we felt just might work. He was given permission to drive the van to school and then on to the farm and home at the end of the day, provided he kept his grades up and actually did the work which he was going to be assigned. He was thrilled and agreed to all of our requirements. Now, with a job he loved, being out of doors, making his own spending money, and permission to drive the van, he was grinning from ear to ear with absolute joy! We felt that we were onto something.

Michael kept that job for the entire school year. He worked every day after school, and many times on Saturdays. His entire Spring Break was spent on that tractor planting tobacco. He never complained. The degree of his anger and sullen mood swings did not dissipate, but it did lessen. His violent tendencies seemed to be tamed to a degree. His face was no longer pasty white, but wind-burn gave way to sunburn and a deep tan. His muscles grew as did his stamina. He shared with us that he planned on becoming a farmer when he graduated. He would work with this farmer and save his money to buy a "small farm with a house and a pond" and make his fortune out-of-doors. At last, Michael had a plan!

When we had first moved to this community, Michael had made friends with Jeff, a boy his age in our church whose father was a deacon and whose mother became my friend as well. Jeff did not go to the same school. Instead he attended the county high school in the southern part of our county. They were in the same grade doing many of the same classes and became fast friends rather quickly. Jeff loved the out-of-doors too and they spent some time hunting and fishing. Sunday afternoons they would ride around the county listening to the radio.

Jeff was the opposite of Michael in many ways. He was self-confident and secure in his own skin. He did not believe in "following the crowd" but gloried in finding his own way. He was a loner as well. Perhaps this is why the two of them became so close. At any rate, Jeff was good for Michael. He did not take any bullying from him and did not put up with the anger or sullenness. He would just leave and go home or bring Michael home if they were in his car. Michael eventually learned that to be Jeff's friend entailed some rules thar were not impossible to follow. In fact, they were quite similar to the rules we had at home. Jeff felt comfortable in our home, and we were comfortable with him. These two would be fast friends for the rest of their lives. Distance often separated them, but when they were back together, it was the same relationship. Michael sought Jeff's presence in some hard times of his adult life, and Jeff was always there for him. I have thanked God for bringing Jeff into his life so many times.

Of course, there were other young people in his life as well. Most of them were from our church family. Michael did not care about girls, but he tolerated them in the church group. He realized that they were a part of growing up and managed to cope. Jeff felt much the same way. They had each other. Some of the boys with whom Michael associated were not the ones that we would have selected, but we knew that he had to find his way.

One day, I was changing the sheets on his bed and as I tucked the corner, I felt something under the mattress. When I drew it out, it was plastic wrap in a flat package encasing marijuana! My stomach just flipped! I could not believe it. We had been through so much with Michael, I just could not fathom that he would do this. Of course, when he came in that night, I confronted him and he insisted that he was just "holding it for a friend." Not for a moment did I believe it and I told him that. I also put my foot down with some of his associations and took away the van except for school and work. Naturally, that brought back the anger and sullen moods as well as the bullying of Mark and Charlaine. At that time, marijuana was not as plentiful as it is now, nor was it accepted at all. I did believe that we could nip this in the bud. Little did I know.

We kept close tabs on where he went and with whom for many, many weeks after that. I suppose that is how I figured out that he was smoking. I did all of the laundry and the smell of cigarette smoke was on his clothes from time to time. He insisted that he had been with people who were smoking, but I knew that was just his story. So, we sat down with him again and explained that if he wanted to have another good season of football, he needed to take better care of his body.

We got through the junior year of high school with no more major episodes and he went back to work for the summer. He was proud of his job and of the fact that he would be back on the football field again in the fall for his senior year. He had begun to date and even gone to the prom with a girl from our church. He insisted that "it did not mean a thing" but he seemed to be maturing and not so different from others his age. This was a relief.

His senior year of high school began. He had passed all of his classes his junior year and had accumulated enough credits that he would only be in school for half days which would put him back in the fields for more hours each day. Of course, he would have to leave earlier to get to football practice, but he did not mind that. He had found himself when he found football, for sure.

His senior year football season began. Mark was playing now as well. They were on the starting team together. The first game was an away game, so we had traveled to the town with Charlaine to see them play. They were expected to win this game and both boys were excited. When they came onto the field, I was so excited for them. I could not help but think of them as those little babies to whom I had given bottles and changed diapers and taught them to speak and to walk. Now here they were all grown up.

The first series of the game we had possession of the ball. Since Michael was defense, he was not on the field; however, since Mark was on offense, we watched him play his first game as a high school varsity player. All was well.

When the other team got the ball and Michael went onto the field, he looked so big. The first play from scrimmage there was a pile-up at midfield. We were on our feet in the stands when we saw the coach and the medic run onto the field. The next thing we saw was that the player on the ground was Michael.

Even when they were playing little league, both boys had warned me that if they were ever down they did not want to look up and see my face looking down at them. I was told in no uncertain terms that mother or not, I was not to come onto that field. My heart was in my throat, and I wanted so badly to run out there and help my son. But, I did not think that my legs would take me.

The next thing we saw was Michael being helped to his feet and carried off of the field by two of his teammates. He was holding one leg in a bent position and I just knew that was not good. They propped him on the bench and the medic began to work on him. I begged my husband to go and find out what was what. The game began again and I saw Mark go over to the bench and bend over to talk to Michael then look up at us with a look of concern.

When the medic motioned for Charles to come to the bench, I wanted to go too but was sent back to my seat. I could only watch and wait. Michael was moving, but he was not getting up.

Charles came back to tell me that Michael had "torn his knee up." One of the players for the other team had fallen on his extended leg and it twisted severely. Needless to say, he did not go back into the game. We wanted to put him into the car and take him on back to the hospital but the coach told us that he would have to ride the bus. I was furious. But, I had learned the hard way that when it comes to football, Mothers have NO say.

We met the bus at the school and took Michael straight to the hospital where he was x-rayed and treated. The diagnosis was that he had torn his knee and would need surgery. There would be many days and nights of pain and unhappiness, of anger and bitterness, or sullen spells, and despair beyond any we had ever imagined for him. We learned that anger is often symbolic of one's feelings toward himself and others. He felt hard toward the boy who had hit him, toward school in general, toward the world at large. Perhaps he felt that we had let him down in some way. We would never know.

Surgery was scheduled at a Sports Medicine facility in another city with the doctor for the Atlanta Falcons—our professional football team. Michael came home in a cast from his hip to his toes. The recovery began with weeping and wailing—and that was just me. Michael was in constant pain and discomfort. He was out of school for the last two weeks before Christmas and then Christmas holidays. There would be no trip to grandmother's house for Christmas. Instead, he and I would stay home by the fire and do our best to improve his spirits.

Years later, Michael confided to me that when he came out of the anesthetic in the hospital and was given strong pain meds, he said to himself, "Where have you been all of my life!"

That was it—the beginning of the end of a "normal life" for Michael. Oh, he went back to school on crutches, finally got the cast off and went to physical therapy and rehabilitation. He dated. He even had a regular girlfriend and they decided that they would neither of them see anyone else. She was his prom date. A very nice girl, we welcomed her to our home. He would go and get her and bring her to church on Sunday nights and then to supper at our house.

His grades suffered. Of course, he could not work. All that he could see for himself was more pain medicine and more pain and nothing to do. There was a lessening of control for him as he surrendered to his fate and lost all hope.

Graduation week came and we did not know if he was going to graduate or not until the afternoon of the graduation ceremony! There was a party after graduation and he and his girlfriend were to attend. At the ceremony he looked so angry and so sullen. There was no smile at all. He shuffled across the stage to receive his diploma and there was no joy whatsoever. After the ceremony he brought his diploma to us and went off to the party. We looked at one another wondering what would be next for our Michael.

Well, it was not good.

Shortly after graduation, he broke up with his girlfriend. That led to depression beyond anything we could have imagined. He got into fights, some of which he started himself. One evening he came home bloody and angry. He had discovered that his ex-girlfriend was dating another guy and had run him off the road where they had fought on the highway. That led to a showdown with the parents of the girl, with the sheriff, and a very long night of listening to him rave and rant about the hand life had dealt to him and why he could not be like everyone else.

He was back at work and had been since the Spring but even that did not give him the solace he needed. Jeff had left to join the Navy which left Michael without his best friend and at loose ends for what came next.

Chapter Nine

Seeking a Future

Michael had wanted to join the Air Force and had gotten as far as going to South Carolina for his intake physical when the doctors discovered how badly his knee was damaged. He was turned down and sent back home.

Needless to say, he was a broken young man. From his earliest years he had been enamored with airplanes. As a child he would watch the crop dusters over the fields of cotton where we were living. One day he even rode his bike to the small landing strip the crop dust pilots used to refuel and load their chemicals. The pilots sort of "adopted" him because they saw his enthusiasm. One of the pilots even let him sit in the cockpit of the plane and we took his picture. That was among Michael's most treasured possessions from his early childhood through the time of his death.

As a young adult he had his heart set on being in the Air Force and often told us that even if he only got to work on the planes, he would be happy just to be around them. We took him to all of the air shows that were within driving distance of our home and when he was old enough, he and Jeff would go to the shows and spend the day with the planes.

So, to have that dream come to a screeching halt was demoralizing for him.

His next goal was to become a crop dust pilot. After talking with the local pilots, he got information about the training required, where he would have to go, how long it would take and the cost. This goal was not beyond his reach, but he had to be twenty-one years old to enter the school, and he was only eighteen.

Continuing to work on the farm and hanging out with some of his friends from the football team and from our little town, he was not in the best frame of mind. His anger issues were still paramount with regard to the breaking up with his girlfriend and the chip on his shoulder had grown significantly with his failure to get into the Air Force.

Having been offered a scholarship in Art to attend a junior college supported by our State Baptist Convention, he decided to "give it a try." Michael was a gifted artist. From his childhood drawings through high school, he had been in demand among his peers to illustrate programs and make posters. He loved drawing planes and had always filled his notebooks with drawings from tiny prop planes to modern jets. So, he accepted the scholarship to our surprise and off to college he went.

Our surprise was largely the result of his basic dislike for school at all levels from learning to read to high school algebra. He had never been happy in school, often literally resenting having to go. So, for him to want to go to college was surprising but thrilling at the same time. We reasoned that perhaps the drawing would keep him interested and allow him to "find himself." We gave our full support in preparing him and getting him there and settled into his dorm room. When we left the campus, we wanted to take a deep breath, but there was more hope than anything else.

Our prayers continued.

Chapter Ten

Escalation

While the exodus from our home to a college dorm for Michael brought some much-needed calm to our daily routine, this was not the case for our lives overall. Mark and Charlaine went about their school and home lives with less turmoil, that was for sure; but, there was always a tense undercurrent about what was really going on and how long this would last. The answer came rather quickly and not too smoothly.

Michael began to show up in my classroom—I was teaching in a large high school located between the college where Michael was now living and our home. Thinking that he was just a little anxious about the new life of independence and decision-making, I welcomed him, introducing him to my class and urging him to take a seat and wait until I had a break so that we could chat.

He wanted none of that. He wanted to chat with me immediately and resented the fact that the students were "looking" at him. What else could he expect? He had come into their classroom as a stranger who was very familiar with their teacher. The school year was still young and they were not even accustomed to me yet—nor I to them. So this presented a very uncomfortable scene for me. Michael seemed to have no real reason for coming and just sort of hung around until a break between classes gave me a chance to talk to him. He shared that he just wanted to see me and tell me that everything was fine. I sensed that there was some sort of tension just under the surface but knew that he would not respond to questioning so I just backed off as my next class entered the room. Michael stayed for another half hour or so and waved goodbye and was gone.

That afternoon on my way home I tried to make sense of what had happened and put it into perspective. He did not ask for money: indeed, when I offered it, he turned it down. He did not appear to be troubled but there was some sort of anxiety, particularly about the students. Not knowing what to do or how to handle it, I went home and shared it with my husband who was disappointed that I had allowed him to stay in the classroom rather than sending him on his way. However, knowing that Michael was truly lacking in self-confidence, I had not wanted to add to that by brushing him off.

He came back to my classroom periodically just like that. On some of the visits he would bring a friend to whom I would be introduced and they would hang out for an hour or so and then be gone. When he came home and we had some time where he felt comfortable, I asked him about these visits. He took my questions to mean that I did not want him there, that I was "ashamed" of him, that I just wanted "to be rid" of him. At length he even said, "You just sent me to school to be rid of me, I know." I was stunned.

At school, he was doing quite well. He was excelling in his art studies and had several pieces entered in the show in the early Spring. Obviously, he loved the art classes but was enjoying psychology as well. Eager to share all that he had learned, he was busily "interviewing" his siblings at the end of the class. His English classes were quite successful as well. We shared the opinion that perhaps he had found himself in college. He liked his roommate and was staying on campus on the weekends to work on his art. We were thrilled when his grades came at the end of the year and he had not only passed but done quite well.

During the summer, he worked on the farm again and in the tobacco fields from sunup to sundown but never complained. He did get back with his group of friends from the community and school but things were obviously not as good as we hoped. We suspected that he was drinking and knew pretty well that he was smoking. A conversation with him about both bore no fruit. He was feeling his independence.

But, things were not good at all. Michael had begun to hurt himself. We first realized this when terrible bite marks appeared on his forearms. Questioning him, we got only a simple, "Don't worry about it!" We increased our vigilance and realized that other things were happening too. He scaled himself from his neck to his waist when he removed his radiator cap while the radiator was hot. Later, he had a smashed finger from time to time, and later he even admitted to going to the dentist to get a tooth pulled. All of these things were done so that he would qualify for pain killers when we took him to the doctor.

Yes, we realized that we had a major problem on our hands for in addition to this bizarre behavior he was obviously smoking and drinking. We had a rule in our home that there would be no tobacco nor alcohol at ANY time. He did not break that rule, for he never brought it home, but we spotted the residual effects readily. When confronted he would become very angry and accuse us of not trusting him or believing him. Things were just going from bad to worse despite all of our efforts on his behalf.

One night quite late, we got a telephone call. Michael and Jeff had run off of the road into a ditch in the van and needed to be pulled out. My husband got a chain and he and Jeff's dad went to get them. When he returned, towing the van with Michael steering, he was not happy. Both Jeff and Michael had been drinking. There was some lecturing and then he sent Michael off to bed.

We were up for hours discussing what was happening and what we could and could not do about it. Taking this new behavior into consideration along with the history of anger, disobedience, disrespect, and the fits of depression and anxiety, we were fairly lost in what our roles as parents could really be. He was pretty independent with his job and his schooling with a scholarship, so we had to tread that line pretty lightly. The old "as long as you are under my roof you will do as I say" did not seem to be the way to go.

We knew that Jeff would get the third degree at his home as well. We felt that we could depend on his family to take some sort of action with him that would leave Michael without the argument that we were too strict and the like. The decision was made to be firm when we talked to him the next morning, assuring him that this behavior was not acceptable in our family and that if it continued we would have to do something—we just were not ready to make the decision on what that would be.

The next morning, he was contrite—but clearly simply because he was not sure how much damage was done to the van. We attempted to talk to him about drinking and what alcohol could do and what the consequences of the night could have been. He was having none of it. The resentment of our intrusion into this facet of his life was severe. He was not only angry, he was furious. Our opinions were "old fashioned" and we were "too strict" and "everybody's doing it." But, he did say—not promise, just say—that he would be more careful about his driving.

The van was not damaged, he had just lost control and gone into the ditch. Nothing was even dented. So, he was back in action immediately. While we suspected that he was drinking and smoking the rest of the summer, we had no proof and therefore nothing that we could do. Needless to say, times were most uncomfortable.

When he left the farm to go back to school in the Fall, there was no hesitation at all. He was eager to return to his art classes and we were eager to see what was next. The summer had been relatively uneventful, so we had high hopes for him.

This did not last long. The next thing we knew he had been arrested for fighting at a movie theater in the town where I taught. While he was banged up somewhat, we learned that he and some guys on the baseball team had been drinking and got into a fight among themselves in the parking lot which resulted in two of them going to the hospital and the others to the Sheriff's office.

A hearing was set and although he was now twenty-years-old, we were informed. On the night of the hearing, Charlaine and I went—my husband would not be a part of it. When Michael came into the courtroom and saw us there he was so angry. He looked at us with fire in his eyes. I know that had he been able to get to us, he would have gone into one of his diatribes. I did not want to be subjected to that.

One by one, the boys were called before the judge and stood with their parents before him. The judge was firm in his questioning and looked each one of them in the eye as he sentenced them. When it was Michael's turn, I went with him to the judge and stood quietly as he was questioned. The judge repeated the same words of caution that we had used but added warnings about fighting in public and what types of sentencing that could bring as well as the physical danger. He spoke about alcohol and how it could lead to no good end. This was not a comfortable time. He listed the injuries Michael had incurred and asked if he had been to the hospital. He looked him squarely in the eye and asked him what his plans were for his life. Michael told him about wanting to fly and the judge gave him a nice lecture about alcohol and driving as well as the prohibition that one could not fly a plane and drink. That was as good as gold for me. At length, Michael was given a fine and seven days of community service.

Then it was time for Charlaine and me to face up to Michael and listen to his raving about how he had been mistreated, that the cops did not know that they were doing, that he and his friends were just having a little fun, and why was it that he could not do just as he pleased. He was so angry that his face was red; he was loud and obnoxious; he was threateningly accusatory toward us; he just wanted to "live his life." When he ran out of steam, he got into the van and left.

At home, we spent a sleepless night trying so hard to determine what we were doing wrong and how we could make things better for him. Neither of us could come up with a plan. We reviewed all that the doctors had told us about his emotional problems and the rage that he was harboring against what or whom we did not know. We did know that the road he was beginning to take was not the one that would lead to success. How to handle this and maintain his trust became the mission of our lives.

Knowing that he was at school became both a comfort and a fear. We were glad that he was pursuing his art and doing well in his studies, at least we hoped that had continued, but we were afraid that these new-found "friends" and the prevalence of alcohol in the area might not be the combination that he needed.

Our research and consultation with a doctor on our own led us to believe that this new behavior was clearly just the old behaviors manifesting themselves in a new way. In short, we were handling the same anger, disrespect for authority, depression, and mood swings with which we had been dealing for years. Except, now we were handling them with an adult. We were cautioned that his tendency to violence and the subsequent fights were harbingers of a deep-seated hatred of some type and that the self-loathing which he seemed to carry was a part of that. If he hated himself, why should others think differently was his attitude and demonstrated by his resentment of all authority including ours. Now, since he was an adult, that could lead to disaster.

We had no idea what our role should be much less how to go about handling the situation at all. We were anxious ourselves. However, when the next event came along, we were totally unprepared again.

During his time in college, his deep love for music increased to gigantic proportions. He began to collect the 78 rpm vinyl records. Unlike anything else in his life, he took great care of them, keeping them sorted by genre and artist. He began to lean toward the rock and roll music and had his favorite artists. We learned to buy him records or give him gift certificates for records whenever there was a gifting occasion. He cherished his records.

His stereo system was not the greatest—Santa had brought it to Mark and him years ago. So, for Christmas, Santa brought him a fairly good system which he dearly loved.

But the system he enjoyed the most was the one in the little blue van. He upgraded it constantly and worked on it regularly. He would ride around the area just so he could listen to his music. Often, he would just go out to the garage and sit in the van with the music going. He learned many of the lyrics and he and I discussed them as if they were poetry.

When he realized that we were not going to have problems with his music, he was thrilled. He began to draw illustrations of the lyrics so that they looked like album covers. Music became the strongest force in his life.

With a cousin in the music business, the children had always had access to concert tickets and seen many of the most popular artists. Now, this became of even greater value. Mike saved the ticket stubs and bought the records and cassette tapes of the concerts. His collection was quite precious to him.

He loved Elton John and had every record and tape ever made as well as going to his live concerts. He knew the lyrics to all of the songs. Now, Michael was not a singer—not by any means, but there was something about the rhythm of the music and the words of the artist that spoke to him.

From the age of about ten when he discovered the group Three Dog Night, through his fondness for Elton John, and Blue Oyster Cult, he loved all music. One of his happiest days was when Charlaine was about three and picked out the song “Bad, Bad Leroy Brown” on the piano. Michael was sure that she was a genius.

The fondness of music and the way it spoke to his life was born while Michael was in college. That fondness grew into a real passion and become one of the few things he dedicated himself to preserving. His collection of vinyls went with him each time we moved and remained the object of his most dedicated care.

Chapter Eleven

Fork in the Road

When the school year ended, Michael moved all of his things home and took up his job on the farm. There was an eerie calm about him. His attitude was anxious and he was continually depressed and moody. My thought was that this would be how we would be forced to live for the rest of our lives. That was disturbing.

One of the psychiatrists had warned us several years before that Michael might never be able to live a normal life. Holding a steady job was out of the question. Maintaining a relationship with a woman and having a family would likely be most difficult if at all possible as well. This was daunting to us.

One thing that bothered my husband the most was how the people of our church would view all of this. Would they see us to blame? Would Michael's behavior cast a shadow on his ministry? How would the youth program in our church be affected? Would his reputation as a minister be tainted?

This attitude bothered me so much. How others viewed US was not as important to me. My concern was for Michael himself and how he would be affected physically, mentally and emotionally. I was also concerned for Mark and Charlaine and what all of this might do to them. Michael was already resentful of Mark for his success in school, socially, spiritually, .athletically, and his all-around good nature. His resentment for Charlaine did not seem to be as acute. He was proud of her musical ability and seemed to feel more protective of her, treating her as a sort of "buddy." I wanted to meet the needs of all three of them making no one of them have to suffer because of one of the others. I felt like I was living in a minefield.

Then one day, he came home from the farm and changed his clothes and left again. Hours later, he returned and asked to talk to his father and me. We went to the church where my husband had his office and sat down, just the three of us and he dropped a bomb on us.

All on his own, he had gone to the State Prison located in our county and applied for a job some time before. He had furnished all his materials and they had ordered his college transcript. Today, he had been called back for an interview and hired as a Correctional Officer. He would leave for training in ten days.

We were stunned. First of all, he had done all of this on his own without our knowledge at all. He had just turned twenty-one, so he was legally an adult and did not need our permission. We had not been prepared for him to take responsibility for himself. After all of the warnings from doctors over the years, we had felt that we would be the ones responsible for him all of his life. But, he had proven us wrong.

Then, neither Charles nor I had ever thought of his going into Criminal Justice. After all, Michael had so much disrespect and resentment for authority that we would have thought that would be the last place he would ever want to spend his life working. But, he had proven us wrong and taken it upon himself to find himself a career.

We were proud of him. Both of us expressed our pride in him and he seemed to respond to that. He told us all about the training and all that would be required of him. We felt that the physical requirements of the boot camp would not be a problem since he had stayed in good physical shape working on the farm so much. We told him that and it earned us a great, big smile. He told us that his college transcript had exempted him from some of the academics and that made him smile again.

Then, I did a stupid thing. I asked him what about his art. He ducked his head and I knew that I had done the wrong thing. He told us that in high school when he was doing a mural for the school that some of the guys had made fun of him, telling him that art was for "queers." While he was in college, the guys in his dorm and the baseball players had bullied him saying that if he was an artist, he must be gay. That had ended his dream of having a studio and drawing for a living. My heart just broke. First of all, the knowledge of the pain he had undergone at the behest of these guys—his friends—hurt me deeply. Knowing that he had handled it alone hurt even more. But, realizing that this God-given gift likely would never be realized made me sad.

He went into some detail about the weapons for which he would be trained. Having always held a deep respect for guns, now the idea of actually being allowed to use one seemed to be most attractive to him.

He was happy. He seemed to be about to do something that made him pleased with himself. That was a whole new emotion for him. Realizing that gave me a sense of comfort that I had not known for a very, very long time. Yes, he would be working in a maximum-security prison but he would be trained for that job which seemed to please him. So, we congratulated him again and relaxed in the glow of self-esteem that seemed to be setting up within him. How we hoped that this was the answer he had been seeking.

Shortly thereafter, we learned that we would be changing church fields. After six years we would now be moving about 250 miles away. Our first thought was for Michael. These fears proved unfounded, he had it handled.

When he realized that we were moving, he had made arrangements to move into a house with one of his friends who also worked at the prison. They would share the utilities and Michael would pay him rent. He would have his own room which he would furnish with the furniture from his room in our house. He seemed so excited over this new move of independence and accepted all of the responsibility with glee.

So, we helped him to move and get himself settled then off we went to another church field.

Mark would be beginning college so this move was really just the two of us and Charlaine who was in high school.

Our nest was beginning to empty. We had made some general plans about what we would do when the children moved on, but now that it was about to happen, we found ourselves a bit hesitant.

A year passed! Everything was going nicely. Charlaine liked her new school; Mark was settled in college with a new group of friends and a new goal in life; Charles was busy as could be in his new pastorate; and, I had a new job that was most interesting.

Then, the bomb dropped.

A phone call during dinner told us that Michael had been "seriously injured" at the prison and had been hospitalized in a large city on the coast. The information was sketchy. We began to try to get the details. What we learned rocked us to the core of our souls and changed the lives of our family forever.

Michael had been taken hostage by a prisoner on death row. This man had held him in a stairwell for hours during which time he had assaulted him over and over, raping him repeatedly, cutting his throat shallowly thirteen times, breaking his back, and slamming him into the concrete to further damage his bad knee and break the other one as well. When Michael had been rescued at last, he had been taken to a local hospital and "patched up" before being moved to the city where he was in the psych ward. The information that we got was more than two weeks old. Michael had experienced a total emotional breakdown in addition to the physical injuries and had been hospitalized for that. We were told that we should not visit him until further notice.

Our pain was beyond comprehension!

There was nothing that we could do.

That was when it hit me. My children were now adults and as such, they had their own lives, responsibilities and the like. I was not prepared for that. For so many years, I had shouldered those responsibilities and was accustomed to their coming to me with their aches, pains, problems and the like. Now, they were ready to take those on for themselves—and if they were not ready, the time was here for Michael at least.

We were concerned for Michael. Our minds went back to what the doctors had told us about his becoming an adult and the likely problems that would arise. That was when we learned that, in all probability, there was some nerves or the like that had never quite developed in Michael's brain. One of the doctors had opined to us that in all probability there were some of the network that did not connect at all and others that were cyclical. We wondered if he could handle what had happened. Then, we came to the realization that whether he could or could not, this situation had been thrust upon him.

This was a time of great testing for my faith. I prayed to God for answers as to why this had happened to Michael. He had been through so h much in his young life that he certainly did not need such a horrendous thing to happen to him just as he was beginning to find a path that he enjoyed walking. I prayed. We prayed as a family. We wanted answers, yes, but more than that, we prayed for God to keep Michael safe, to touch his soul as well as his body, and to keep him strong. Yes, during these long, dark hours, my faith was tested. We drew even closer to God as we cast this burden—our son—on Him, confident that His will would be done.

Two days later, we were allowed to talk to him by telephone. He sounded so small and sad. I could only see him as that little boy I had known and my heart just broke again. He told us that he was alright and that he would be coming up to visit us as soon as possible and that we should not be worried.

Fat chance!

Our prayers and our hearts went out to him. We wondered at how he really was. We opined to one another that he was being strong for us and that was a turn of the tables. We wondered if this would break him mentally, if he was strong enough to handle the emotions. We had no answers, just fears and hopes.

Released from the hospital, he and his roommate went to Florida for some R and R. This initially upset me. I felt that if he left the hospital, he should have come home; however, his roommate—whom we all loved and trusted completely—called and made me aware of the fact that Michael was not ready to see us yet. He had to make sense of what had happened to him and how it was going to affect him for the rest of his life. Also, because Michael had always been so conscious of what other people thought of him—even with a phobia that people were always looking at him wherever he went, hence his reluctance to be in crowds—now he felt that people would be looking at him and judging him even more so. With this explanation, I tried to calm down.

When he returned from that little "vacation," he went to visit Mark at college. Mark shared with us that he saw Michael in the hall of the dorm and had not been expecting to see him. Going up behind Michael, Mark tapped him on the shoulder and Michael turned around ready to fight, his face contorted with sheer anger and rage. That is how "trigger happy" he had become. The slightest little act that was not expected or routine would set him off. Mark spent the weekend listening to Michael and reassuring him.

By the end of the summer he was released to come to our house on Workman's Compensation. He could not handle going to work at the prison and being in the presence of the convict who had damaged him so badly. When he drove up our drive I was overcome with emotion and the fears were back. We greeted him with hugs and kisses and he allowed us to fawn over him a little. He was so thin, and so pale. He was jumpy and anxious over every little thing. He picked at his food and wanted a nightlight in his room to sleep.

In the ensuing weeks we would see the grown-up Michael return to the adolescent Michael as he experienced emotional highs and lows as he attempted to gain his strengths. What a rollercoaster this was!

Always an eager reader, he began to read constantly. I would take him to the Public Library where he would choose an armload of books to read at home in his room alone. He read books about violent crimes, jihadists, various religions, crime stories, war books, and airplanes. We made least one and often two trips a week to the library. When we were at my little mountain house, he read so voraciously that he totally read everything in that library about these subjects. He visited that library so often that people thought he worked there. Magazines were also interesting to him. He kept up with what was going on in the world by reading the weekly news magazines and newspapers as well as all gun and crime magazines.

As an English teacher, I did not approve of his obsession with these types of reading material, but he had no interest in novels: he did expand his interests to history, especially military history.

After some time, he bought a television set for his room. He would stay awake all night long watching crime shows and The History Channel. NASCAR was one of his obsessions: he never missed a race and worshipped Dale Earnhardt. He also watched football any time that it was on—any team, any day, even reruns. Baseball and Basketball held no appeal to him whatsoever.

And, eating! He ate constantly. Often at mealtimes, he would pick at his food and at times, not even eat at all. Then, he would make trip after trip to the refrigerator. I learned to stock up on the snacks that he liked—string cheese and Lorna Doone cookies were his favorites—and to cook extra and fix small containers of left overs for him to microwave during the night or the day when I was gone. There was never any food wasted at our house while Michael was there. His most favorite food of all was ice cream—vanilla. I could not keep enough of it on hand for him. Often I would come home to an empty carton still in the fridge, often with the spoon inside.

Mark came home from college for the Christmas holidays and they were back to sharing a room. This had good points as well as not-so-good points. They talked late into the night—that was good. They argued over tiny, little things and great big enormous things. Our home became a battlefield one moment and a love fest the next. Charlaine was caught in the middle of it, but she could retreat to her room. Charles and I became the referees which was not a pleasant job.

Christmas was rather uncomfortable. We tried very hard to have our "normal Burgess Christmas." However, this was not to be. Michael resented the preparations for Christmas and the activities in which we were involved both at my school, our church, in the community and with Charlaine. Mark got a part-time job for the holidays and that gave Michael some problems—he was not working, could not work and felt that this put him in a negative light.

The discomfort that each of our family felt for Michael was palpable. We so regretted what had happened to him, but we so wanted him to know that we still loved him and that life would go on and this too would pass away. He could not, or would not see that.

When Mark went back to school we anticipated peace and quiet. This was not to be. Michael was unable to settle down. He would sleep all day and be up all night. Charlaine would be gone to school, Charles and I would be at work and he would get into his car and be gone when we got home. We never knew where.

At length, we realized that he had found a place to hang out that was known for strippers, drugs, and alcohol. He was an adult and forbidding him to go there was out of the question. His resentment of us as authority figures was back. Anger, disrespect, hate, violence, profanity—all of the things we hated so much in him—were back. He did not come home drunk, but he came home angry because he was doing what he wanted and knew that it was wrong so it made him mad. The battlefield was back.

One really good thing came out of hanging out in this area though. He discovered the airport there. This was a small airport that handled much of the private traffic that would have been handled by the large metro airport nearby; however, it was also utilized by many of the private plan owners in the area and—most of all, and best of all for all of us—they had a flying school. When Michael discovered this, he began hanging out with the pilots and instructors there. He learned a great deal about planes and would come home delighted with his day and the new-found knowledge. We were thrilled! He had something to occupy him mentally and challenge him as well. At length, he made the decision to learn to fly!

This was both thrilling and disturbing to us. Because of his nervous condition, problems with instruction, and least of all a wonder at how his brain was really affected, we did not know whether to encourage or discourage. We elected to encourage him. He was so happy and so dedicated. He threw himself into the lessons. The change in his demeanor was wonderful. He would come home so exhilarated that he would go on and on and on about the controls, the principles of aviation and all that he had learned. Poring over his books late at night, we saw the shadow of the "old Michael" returning. This improved over the weeks of his training.

On the day that he was to solo, I confess that I was terrified; however, seeing the glow in his face and the joy of anticipation, I encouraged him. Charles went with him to witness the flight. I could not go. I was far, far too afraid. When I came in from school that day, I found two excited men. Michael had done it! He had his log bok for me to see, and, proudest of all, he had the cutoff t-shirt signed by the instructors which I discovered was a real trophy.

There would be many dark days ahead for Michael during his lifetime, but he hung onto that log book and that t-shirt with all of the pride in the world. This became his touchstone. When things were really bad for him, and he felt his life falling apart, he would always say, "But I can fly a plane! I learned to fly! I have proof!"

When Michael died, Mark took that log book and t-shirt and holds it in the high esteem that Michael did. Truly, for all of us this was a monumental achievement.

He made a trip back south to visit his friends. We had two weeks of peace and he was back filled with more vitriol than when he left. Recuperating from that trip took almost two weeks during which time we wondered how and even if we could survive.

During that trip, he met a girl who apparently made the overtures and with whom he became intimately "involved." She called him regularly and when he would be at his lowest, he would call her. Claiming that he really had no feelings for her, that she was "just a friend," and that she liked him but he did "not like her like that," he continued to talk with her and she wound up coming to see him several times. Each time he returned south, he would "date" her and they grew closer and close. Still he vowed that there was "nothing there."

Not until he left for Michigan did this relationship fizzle out. When Michael got himself "cleaned up" she was part of the past. Of course, we had been suspicious all along that she was a part of his addiction problems. When there was no longer any contact, we realized that more than likely, we had been right.

His days became filled with meaningless activities that led him to people who were willing to use his inability to be fiscally responsible and supply him with whatever he wanted without thinking about the results. Again, he began to show up in my classroom for no reason at all and just want to hang around and challenge the students who might "look" at him. There are no words to describe the uneasiness and discomfort in our home.

We tried to interest him in the activities of home by encouraging him to help with the yard work, or with the house work. He hated being "told" to wash the dishes or mow the grass; but, occasionally, I would come home to find the kitchen immaculate, the dishes washed, dried and put away and on some occasions the floors vacuumed, laundry done and supper begun. This was very infrequent, but it did happen. He would ride the lawnmower to cut the grass because "no one bothered" him while he was doing this. He kept his car washed and cleaned out but his room was more often than not an absolute wreck! There was no way of anticipating what mood we would encounter on a given day nor what we might see unfold.

I had inherited a little house up in the mountains when my mother died. I used it for the family in the summer and occasional weekends. I approached Michael about going up there and setting up housekeeping and staying there. He would have no expenses; there would be peace and quiet; he would have unlimited time for television viewing and could osleep as much as he wanted. The only rules that I made was that he could not smoke in the house: I feared a fire.

He was so happy. He would have his own place and be able to prove himself to us. So, Mark came home from college and helped him move his stereo, clothes and books up to the house. Michael was all set up – or so we thought.

Before too long, he was bored. He did not know anyone and was not willing to get out and make some friends through the church or our relatives there. He shared with me that he had gone to town and bought a "six-pack" and then in the grocery store found two young women and asked them to come home with him. They did. Apparently, they "listened to music" and drank the beer before leaving to go home. I was stunned!

In this tiny little town, he had found a way to continue his indulging ways. Later, I would learn that he also found someone to supply him with a "meager supply" of the drugs he preferred. Upon acquiring this knowledge, I did some investigating and confronted the pharmacist who had filled his bogus prescription. Continuing my observations, I determined that this was not unusual for this store. With my complaints and reports, that store closed!

Tiring of the rural life of the mountains, he came back to our house and with Mark's help, moved his stereo back as well. This experiment in him living on his own and working through some of the emotional problems like he had thought he could do did not work at all!

Weeks turned into months and he finally decided to go back to work. He was put on a different shift and he went back to the house where he had been living. We hoped for the best. This lasted almost a month and he had a total breakdown on duty and was shipped to the hospital again. He was in psychiatric rehabilitation for several months and then allowed to return to us.

The result was more of the same. We were not living, we were existing.

One night he was watching a football game in his room and came out into the hall to speak to me and began to fall into the wall and slide down to the floor with his eyes turned up into his head and shaking all over. He was out cold. The EMTs were summoned and brought him out of unconsciousness. We were all terrified. They administered care and told us that he was just overly stimulated with the game as far as they could tell. They encouraged us to check back with our doctor.

This happened twice more. Trying to determine what was wrong and what all of this meant, we realized that each time this happened, he had just returned from a trip South to visit his friends where we suspected that he had done some drugs and drank more than enough alcohol. Not that we approved, we did not; however, the time had come when we were seeking answers any way that we could find them.

Michael went right back to the same behavior as before. He was hanging out during the day and in the evenings totally out of control. His language to Charlaine was disrespectful and, at times, downright profane. Mark was away at school, so she bore the brunt of his anger. He resented being at home and not having his "own place." He wanted to go back to work but feared that he would never be able to do that. The scenery was the same day in and day out. Nothing pleased him. He would not go to church. All he wanted was to hang out.

By this time, we were sure that he was not only doing alcohol and smoking but was doing drugs as well. He was mandated by the State, as a part of his Workman's Compensation package, to see a psychiatrist once a week who would report back to the prison system. He kept those meetings up and would come home from each one even more fired up. What went on in those meetings we never learned but he was often angry after them. Occasionally he would have a day when he was morose and moody and just wanted to be left alone, but most of the time it was violent anger and loud lashing out.

In our counseling sessions, we were told that he was more than likely mentally ill and that the emotional turmoil of the hostage event had driven him into manic episodes. We were also told that the continual use of alcohol and drugs was compounding his problems.

His doctor elected to put him on anti-depressants which were supposed to calm his moods; however, they did just the opposite. He was unable to sit still to read a book or to view a television program much less a movie. Viewing football games was interrupted by manic outbursts and angry confrontations. When the meds were stopped, his behavior continued to be moody and anti-social. We were at a loss as to how to act in our own home.

Chapter 12

Family Catastrophe

When he had been on Workman's Compensation for two years, living with us, seeing his psychiatrist once per week, and wallowing in self-pity indulging himself with alcohol and drugs, we learned that my husband had cancer. By the time it was discovered and diagnosed it had spread from his kidneys to his lungs and the doctors gave him six months to live. This shook Michael to his core.

Michael's first reaction was to become resentful and even more belligerent than before. He left the house and we did not see him for almost three days. When he finally returned, he had been on a real bender – alcohol and we never knew what kind of drugs nor where he went. He was totally freaked out.

We were so concerned about him. We had hunted him all over the area with no luck at all. We had called his friends down South where he had lived and visited, all to no avail. Of course, we expected the worst! He could not understand why we had been upset. He was exhausted and totally in the midst of a downward spiral.

He had no idea whatsoever of the tremendous concern this had caused all of us. Instead, he was only concerned about the fact that God was taking his father and he could not deal with it. We attempted to reason with him, to offer all kinds of counseling and to explain that we all needed to make the most of the time that Charles did have left. I was even perfectly honest when I told him that adding another layer of concern right then was not helping but was hindering, that we needed him to be available, clear-headed and sober to offer solutions not more problems. That seemed to catch his attention.

He showered, shaved, ate some wholesome food, and then asked to talk to us. He apologized for his behavior and tried to explain that he just could not handle it; but, if we really believed that he could help, he was ready to do it and would promise to mend his ways. He seemed so sincere that we took him up on it.

Because Michael was home during the day, he agreed to take Charles to chemo. This seemed to stabilize him. He took this errand seriously. He would be solicitous of him and so careful loading him into the car and staying right beside Charles, as if he was trying to endure the pain for or with him. At home he was kind and comforting in every way. He ran errands, helped with meals and cleaning up. He did the laundry and washed dishes. He took pride in his room and even changed the sheets on all of the beds and went grocery shopping.

We saw a whole new side of Michael. I wonder if he realized that we were in crisis and that he could help. He knew that we had been in crisis before with him, and he had only added to that problem. But, when the crisis was happening to his father he determined to be a part of the solution not the problem. He would stay with Charles all day being sure that his meds were given properly and that all of his needs were met. When I would come in from work, he would report to me with a rundown of all that had gone on and question what he could now do to help me.

Much to my absolute surprise, when he had come home to stay with us, he was able to find a supplier of the drugs he preferred almost immediately. Even today, years and years after the fact, I do not know how he did it. In a town where he knew absolutely no one, he found a pusher and began using again. He did not think that we knew that he was using, but it was obvious to us. His demeanor would be quieter, he was never hungry at mealtimes but snacked all night, sleeping was impossible for him. In short, there was no way that we could not know, but he thought that he had us snowed.

I was very up front with him, I told him that he must NOT take any drugs nor drink any alcohol while he was alone with his father. I could not bear the thoughts of Charles needing something and Mike in a stupor totally of no help at all. I was at school all day and Charlaine was at school, so I had to trust him. I told him all of that, and he gave me his word that he would stay clean for Charles.

I believe that he did. Charles would tell me how Michael would bring his meds to him, prepare his lunch, help him to the bathroom, and help him get into the shower and stay right there in the bathroom while he showered. Michael helped him dress saw to it that he was shaven every day and became his personal keeper. We were more than appreciative, we were sure that this was indicative of something good in Michael and that we were getting a real glimpse of hope that he could get better, that maybe all of the counseling was paying off. Apparently, he needed to be needed.

Some weeks into my husband's illness, the doctors shared with us that he was not getting any better despite the treatments and medications, that he had maybe a month left to live. Charles asked that I take him up to the house in the mountains one more time. So, I did. We told the children that they had the weekend off and should do something that they enjoyed.

I drove him up, turned on the heat and got him comfortable before preparing supper. He was not hungry, but I managed to get him to eat a little bit. He fell asleep in the recliner. After a fretful night, I got up and did the chores that needed to be done while he slept. He arose just before noon, and after an attempt at breakfast settled down to watch the World Series.

Of course, he slept through most of it, but he spent a lot of time looking out at the mountains which I had always found very soothing. I think that he did too. That night, he asked that I get paper and pen and he planned his funeral. We discussed the children and what would happen to Michael when the time came. We prayed about it and put the matter into God's hands.

I took a shower and got ready to for bed, then helped him to the shower. I put a stool in the bathtub so that he could sit – he was so weak. Leaving him to enjoy the warm water, I went to turn the bed down when I heard him calling me. When I got there he was hemorrhaging – blood was everywhere, and he was falling. I managed to turn off the water and catch him before he went down, but I was not strong enough to get him out of the tub. Calling 911, I got some help almost immediately. But, by that time he was in shock. My cousin had come when he saw the ambulance and he drove me to the hospital where the doctor told me that Charles was serious and that I should call the children.

Charlaine and Michael were at our house and Mark was visiting his girlfriend in South Georgia. Getting Charlaine on the phone, I told her to come as soon as it was daylight and to bring Michael. She was good at handling him when he would go out of control, and I feared that he would be. She told me that he had gone out with some people and told her that he might not be back that night, but not to worry. She undertook to find him sending her boyfriend out to find his car and see if he could find Michael. Mark was out on the lake night fishing. I left word for him to call immediately when he came in. I told him the same thing: as soon as it is daylight come. He left immediately and came. Charlaine was finally able to locate Michael and get him sobered up to come the next morning.

After meeting with the doctor, we were told that this little mountain hospital could not do what he needed and we should send him back to the hospital near our home by ambulance the next morning. His doctors were there. We took turns sitting with Charles who was so sick that he really did not know what was happening! Michael was a basket case, but he held it together. He listened to all that we had to hear and to say. When decisions were needed, he agreed with whatever we said. He really tried.

Ten days later, Charles passed away.

Summoning the children to the hospital that morning when they told me that he was failing, Michael came first. He had showered and came into the room with a look of total grief on his face. He was trying to be "manly" and strong, but he was like a little boy faced with something he did not understand. He went to his father and for some time just looked down at him. He touched him, and Charles stirred. He did recognize Michael and spoke to him. Michael mumbled back to him with tears in his eyes and choking back sobs. He stood there holding his father's hand until Charlaine arrived. At that time, he moved to the other side of the bed and just kept his eyes glued on his father.

At length Mark came. Charles recognized each of them as they entered and spoke to each of them as well as touched them. We held hands and prayed for strength as we watched life leave the head of our household. Emotions were so strong that we were just so full that no one could speak nor move. The nurse came into the room and turned off the machines telling us that "hearing is the last thing to go, keep talking to him." So we did. One by one we chatted.

Michael took his turn and it was all that he could do to get the words out, but he did.

Then, it was over.

Charles had died!

Our lives as we had known them would be forever changed. That certainly was the harbinger of a new day for Michael.

Our doctor came to sign the death certificate. I noticed Michael follow him out into the hall, but I was so overwrought that I really did not think about it. I would later learn that Michael got a prescription for Xanax claiming severe emotional stress. Needless to say, that bolstered him for the ordeal with which we were all dealing and kept his emotions on a more even level.

We all returned to the house to take care of arrangements and try to deal with our own shock and grief. Six weeks had passed since his diagnosis. Now, he was gone.

Michael went to his room and was alone for a very long time. We let him have his space for we each needed ours as well. In the time leading up to the funeral there was so much to do, and so many people coming and going that there was no time for us to interact with him or to deal with our personal feelings. I did keep my eye on Michael as did Mark and Charlaine. We were careful to include him in any decision and in all of our business. Finally, we had to insist that eat something. . He held up just barely. I just wanted us all to come out of this alive, okay. I wanted Michael to come out of it unscathed, or as together as possible. I suppose that was wishful thinking on my part. How could any of us come out unscathed, much less him with his fragile hold on reality. At times he was sullen and unspeaking: other times he was trying very hard to be cordial

Some friends of his came up for the funeral—his roommate, the girl who liked him so much, and some others. That helped Michael. He felt like he had someone upon whom to lean, I suppose. After the graveside service, we all went back to our house. Each of the children had friends with them and there was plenty of food. Michael asked me if it would be alright if he went to the hotel with his friends and for supper and perhaps spend the night. I looked at him and in his eyes I could see a plea to let him get away from all of the people and the expressions of prayers and the like. I knew that he had stood up about as long as he could and that he was about to collapse, so I agreed.

He packed a few things and left. I did not see him for two days. Charlaine returned to school and Mark went back to his job at the college. When Michael came in, I could tell that he had been drinking and/or drugging as well as being with his friends. I was in no condition to begin a session about his slipping. I just welcomed him home. I think that surprised him.

The ensuing time was filled with settling affairs. Because we lived in the pastorium of the church, we had to find a place to live. The Board of Deacons were very generous allowing us to stay until we could find a place. But, I knew that they needed the house so that they could prepare for the next pastor and made it my number one task to find a house. Mark and Charlaine helped me to look and slowly we realized what we needed, what we wanted, and what we could afford. Charlaine and I found just the house we needed – the room, the location, the style all fit our plans. The bank helped me to arrange a loan and I took Michael to see it. He could not believe that we would have our own house.

We moved into the house six weeks after Charles had died. Mark came to help us move. Michael helped – not a lot. He was wrestling with all that was happening. He knew that he needed to get a hold on his emotions and get himself back to work. Our lives were changing so fast.

Talking with his psychiatrist, they made the decision that after the first of the year he needed to prepare himself to either return to work for the Department of Corrections or find another career. This was tough for Michael. He had hidden behind the alcohol and drugs and us for so long that stepping back into a world of his own was scary for him.

We talked about it and he admitted that he missed having a place of his own. We also talked about the way he had handled the responsibility of his father and how that showed that he likely was ready to take on responsibility again. He brought up his fears, his doubts, and what he felt were the barriers to him going back to a life of his own. We discussed each one of them, and came up with a way to handle them.

At length, he arranged to return to work at another facility – not the one where he had been taken hostage. He actually got excited about going back to work in a new place.

To help him prepare to go back to work, we went shopping for some new clothes. This was a nightmare! We had made a list of all that he needed and wanted and I promised him that we would do this efficiently and get out of there as quickly as possible.

We came to the jeans department and found the style and size that he wanted; but, he refused to try them on. Remember now, he had not worked in almost two years and had been on a steady diet of eating everything and then nothing, of snacks, and pills, and no sleep to all sleep. So, there had to be a difference in his size, but he refused to try on the clothes. To make it even worse, he was sure that every customer in the store and every clerk was watching him. Finally, I gave up and agreed with him that we would just buy things and get out of there.

When we got home, he still refused to try on the clothes. Instead, he washed them all. THEN, he tried them on. The jeans did not fit! (I am not sure that they would have fit before he washed them, but that was beside the point.) In total dismay, I told him to just put them aside and we would decide what to do the next day. Then, unbeknownst to me, he called the store and explained that the clothing did not fit but that he had washed all of it and they told him to just bring it all back and they would refund the money or he could get another size! Imagine that! He was thrilled. So, the next day we repeated the process, but this time, he tried on the clothes.

Shopping was and would always be a nightmare for him!

He went downstate to look over the place of work and the town. I offered to go with him as did Mark and Charlaine, but he wanted to do this for himself. So, he did. To our very pleasant surprise, he liked the facility, the town, and the people and even found a cute little garden apartment. He arranged to move his furniture in and to purchase a washer and dryer as well as some of the things he wanted to have.

He was so proud of himself. Within two weeks, he was ready to move down and go to work. Loading his stereo, his books, and his clothes, he went back into the real world.

Chapter Thirteen

Back to Work

Having Michael go back to work and leave us to move 250 miles south gave me some very strange feelings. I was thrilled to know that he felt well enough to return to work but, I knew that his problems still existed. I prayed diligently that this return to structure as well as the need to become involved and participate would be the genesis of a serious move forward. I also found some confidence in the fact that he would be in a facility that was peopled with minor offenders rather than the capital offenders who had been his charges. Having heard his satisfaction with the warden whom he immediately liked gave me some hope that his resistance to authority might get a working over as well.

All of his reporting back to us was positive. He was so happy to have his own place again. This was his first time to live alone—previously he had shared a house with a friend and another correctional officer. Now, he was on his own. He loved it. He set himself up with furniture and appliances to afford him a comfortable home. He liked his new job. A couple of the other officers he had met in his previous facility and he began to make other friends.

The demands of the job at this new place were totally different. The nature of the facility to house minor offenders was far more relaxed than the tension Michael had lived with when he worked Death Row.This seemed to appeal to him and all of his reports gave us cause to hope.

As the months went on, his calls became fewer and less often. The first hint of problems came when I received a letter from a woman telling me that she and her two children were living with Michael and how much in love they were as well as how eager she was to meet me and get to know me. The letter went on to tell me that they were making a life together and a home together. The obvious clues led me to believe that they were going to marry. I became suspicious, perhaps cautious is a better description of my feelings. I debated what to do.

The next time Michael called me, I mentioned the letter and her name. He became furious. Apparently, the "love affair" was all in her head. Yes, she and her two children were staying with him because she was the ex-wife of one of his "friends" and had nowhere to go. He was befriending her, he said. Somehow, I knew that there was more to this story than I was getting from either of them. I remembered that Michael was a grown man, on his own, and prayed that he knew what he was doing.

A friend from our former church was in the area and went to see Michael reporting back to me that he was heavily into alcohol and drugs again. Further, he told me that the woman living with him was his supplier and was so hooked on cocaine herself that she had lost custody of her children and was actually hiding from the law. This sent all kinds of alarms off in my head.

I debated for a long time about what to do. My prayers ascended for help from God above for I was at a loss. I had visited a support group for families of drug addicts before, so I went back and began to attend the meetings in an effort to understand better how to proceed.

Where I had waited for Michael to call me before, thinking that I was giving him his space, I began to call him weekly. I made it clear that I was not checking up on him, but that I missed him and was interested to know how things were going. At first, he was very timid and apologetic for not getting in touch with me more often. He talked about his new friends and how they would gather at his place to play cards and watch football games. I could only pray that this was true.

He made it very clear to me that he had "gotten rid of" the woman and her children. He was angry that she had written to me and over and over told me that he had no interest in her. That set my mind on edge. He was being too insistent, I thought. But, I wanted to give him space and let him know that I was there if I was needed and that he was NOT alone.

Shortly after this, he admitted to me that he was drinking again. "Just a few beers with my friends" he told me. He denied that he was back into the pills, and that he was not letting the alcohol take over his life again.

Totally inexperienced with alcohol of any kind, I did not realize that beer can have the same effect as illegal drugs—often worse. I came across a report put out by Drug Strategies which called alcohol "America's most pervasive drug problem." And went on to document the claim. They included alcohol-related deaths which outnumbered drug related deaths four to one. One of the comments I found very troubling was that of the probationers interviewed, four in ten admitted that they were under the influence of alcohol when they committed their crime while only one in ten were under the influence of drugs.

The next thing was that he was having trouble at work. He was not happy with his fellow officers and beginning to doubt the honesty of his warden. This made me more anxious than ever, for this was that old resentment of authority beginning to show up again. I found this to be troubling and tried to discuss it with him. He was determined that he was right and the warden "just has it in for me."

About this time, I read that many people cannot and will never be able to drink in moderation. Instead, they often are involved in DUIs with deaths included, domestic abuse, date rape, binges, and blackouts. These people often celebrate even the smallest things with a six-pack, and decry the pits of life with a six-pack going on to miss out on some really good things because of the effects. Then they go into work hung over with a thick tongue and clumsy fingers and cannot perform their duties. Michael was experiencing all of this. He would work his six days and when he came to his three days off, he would drink himself into a stupor. Then, he was off kilter when he went back to work.

At length, I received a call from the warden himself telling me that Michael had been sent to Colorado for rehab. Seems that he was having trouble at work because he was showing up hungover and was using pills again. He told me about the woman who had been living with Michael and that she was the ex-wife of another officer who had separated from her because she was so heavily into cocaine. He told me that the facility in Colorado specialized in working with Correctional Officers and the stress with which they lived. He assured me that things would be good for Michael and that he would be there until he was deemed fit to return to work.

My heart was broken. I wrote to him and expressed over and over my love and support for him. I sent him art supplies and books as well as baked goods. I kept my letters light and cheery in an effort to show him that I believed in him.

He was there for six weeks after which he returned to work. He did not come home for another six weeks and when he did, I was dismayed in the difference. He had lost weight but he was alert, eating well, and showed no signs of alcohol or drug abuse. I took a deep breath.

Then he dropped the bomb. While in Colorado, he had met a girl. She liked him and he liked her. She was from a city less than 100 miles from me. She had been down to visit him a few times, and they had decided that they were going to move in together. She had been in rehab for drugs and was now clean. He had invited her to come down to my house for the weekend.

I was shocked! He had not been interested in a relationship since high school and now had become involved with someone who apparently liked him right back. He was so happy.

When she walked into my house, I was stunned. She was tall, blonde, slender, fair-skinned, and absolutely beautiful. She was dressed stylishly and had a shy personality. From the beginning, I could see that they were interested in one another and wondered just where this would go.

When they left—him to go south back to work and she to go north back to school and work—I did not know what would happen next. To my surprise, I got a phone call from Michael telling me that he had put in for a transfer to a facility near me and, of course, near her. He was coming home the next weekend and wanted me to go with him to find an apartment and help make arrangements for him to move and for her to move in with him.

Shocked! Stunned! What could I say? What could I do? He was a grown man . . . independent . . . she was a grown woman . . . also independent. I was at a loss for the appropriate reaction. So, I agreed to go with him and help him make these arrangements.

She came down and went with us. I was thrilled for them. They seemed to have their feet flat on the ground and were very careful in looking at places and picking out the things that they liked and did not like. By the afternoon, they had selected a town house with two bedrooms that they both agreed would be home for them. She was going to bring her bedroom furniture and Michael would bring all of his furniture and appliances and they could furnish it easily. We made the trips to get the utilities arranged and set up a time when he would move up there and when she and her mother would bring her things. This was very interesting.

Within a month, they were installed in the home, she had found a job and they were keeping house. He was on an even keel and I realized that her knowledge of the problem and commitment to stay clean might be just the ticket for both of them.

They had been living there about a year when Lora called me to say that Michael had admitted himself to rehab in a facility just a few miles over the state line from their home. She told me that he had gotten back into drugs and some alcohol and was having trouble at work.

My heart just about broke.

He was there for six weeks and returned to work. His visits home became more frequent and he spent more and more time telling me all of the things that were wrong at work. Again, the old problem of authority resentment reared its head. He told me that he was clean and sober but that staying that way was difficult with all of the problems at work.

I insisted that he get himself back with a psychologist to deal with the problems at work before they took him over. He told me that he would look into it. I am not sure that he ever did.

Another year went by and he was definitely using again, I could tell. He would come to my house on his days off and spend his time sleeping and watching TV while I was at school. That was when I learned that things were not going well with Lora either. She had a job in retail and worked some evenings and weekends. That left him on his own and he resented that. She liked pretty clothes and makeup and went to visit her mother from time to time and he resented that. She wanted to go back to school, she was studying nursing, and he was all for that, but at the same time he wanted her with him. We spent hours and hours with him delineating all of the problems with her and me trying to show him ways to handle this.

At length, they split. Apparently it was a joint decision. They had a shouting argument and she threatened to leave and he told her to go, so she did. The next day she came with her uncle and a truck and got all of her things and that was the end of that.

He was destroyed. Although he had been the one to send her away, he did not want her to go, he said. He came to my house and lamented all weekend. Remembering that he had been able to find a drug supplier when he was living with us on Workman's Compensation, I feared that he would go that route again. But, I had to go to school. I had a job and I had to do it.

He decided that he wanted to go back to college and get a degree in Criminal Justice. So, I helped him to apply to a local liberal arts college where he could go to school during the day and keep his job since he worked at night. He would come to my house on the days of his school, attend class and sleep, then go to work. He loved it! He was taking Psychology and really into it. His professor was thrilled with his writings and on all of his tests he made A's. He was happy. He was not using to the best of my knowledge and he was functioning at a high level.

Then one day, I came home from school to find my house disturbed—chairs were turned over, the refrigerator was open, books were pulled out of the bookshelves and there was a general state of disarray. I thought that I had been robbed. I called the Sheriff and told them that I had been robbed. I went upstairs wondering if Michael was asleep. He was not in his room, but more things had been pulled out—clothes were everywhere. The bathroom was a shambles. I went downstairs to my room and the door to the deck was open. I found him there eating a dog biscuit. When I spoke, he turned to me and said, "These are really good!" His eyes were glassy and he was high—really high. At that time, I realized that I had not been robbed—Michael had experienced another episode. There was no other explanation.

The police came and reached the same conclusion. They did go all over the house with me and nothing was missing. Michael was staggering and slurring his words and so out of it that I feared, really feared for him. The suggestion was that the police would take him to the hospital where they had a ward for drug rehab and I would meet them there to make the arrangements to admit Michael.

I was so torn up. I packed a bag with clothes and toiletries a few books and the like and took off for the hospital. He was furious with me. His face was flushed and his eyes hard when he told me "Thank you. I have just lost my job." He was so cold.

I called his work and explained what had happened and they were not surprised at all. Seems that he had been missing lots of work and had been in some scuffles with the other officers as well as contentious with the warden. They were very supportive of his admission to rehab and told me that they would work with me in any way possible.

I shared that with Michael who showed no emotion whatsoever. In fact, he was so cold to my visiting him that I left after a short while. I would learn later that he had been on a binge for a few days and had just lost it after his class. The unique thing was that in class that day he had a test and made 110 on the exam, then came home and remembered nothing after that.

He was taking two kinds of pain killers and an anti-depressant. Where he was getting these I did not know and do not know today. But he had quite a stash when I unpacked his things to wash his clothes. At this time, I did not know what to do. Not only, did I no longer have my husband with whom to discuss this, but by this time, Mark was married and living mid-state, and Charlaine had moved to Texas. I went back to my support group and prayed for help to deal with the problem.

Michael was released after six weeks and wanted to get back to see about "my place." He was deemed ready to go back to work. We discussed his life and how he was living it. He admitted what he was doing was not ideal but also admitted that he did not know what he could do about it.

A month or so later he came to see me and told me that he was having trouble again, but that with the help of a drug counselor he had found help in a Methadone clinic in a nearby town. He was going there once a week and getting medication to last him a week. This was creating a buffer that prohibited him from taking any type of drug or any alcohol at all. I had my doubts but he was insistent that this was what was best for him.

He seemed to be better. Certainly he was looking and acting better. He had an appetite and would come to my house on his days off and work in the yard. We would have long discussions and go out to eat. Things seemed to be going well.

This new plan seemed to be working for him. But, deep down inside, I wondered for how long. I hoped that it would be permanent but all of the information that I found and read about Methadone seemed to indicate that there was still a lot of work to be done before it became the be all end all.

Sure enough, there were problems.

Chapter Fourteen

Transition

Things were going from bad to worse. I had a terrible fall and had surgery with extensive rehab. Michael came to help out and took care of my dog and helped at the house. I could tell that he was using, but hoped that it was just the Methadone. One day, we were going to the library so that both of us could get some books. I could not drive yet, so he was driving us downtown. Happy to be out, I was enjoying the scenery when I noticed that the car was weaving. Looking up, I saw that Michael was sound asleep! Asleep driving an automobile in downtown traffic with me as a passenger just talking along.

Frantic, I grabbed the steering wheel to avoid going into the other lane and called out to him. Startled, he shook himself awake and realizing what was happening, took over with a sheepish grin on his face. Needless to say, we stopped as soon as possible and I took over the driving, doctor's advice or no.

We discussed what was happening to him, and he convinced me that it was "just the Methadone." Alarmed, I begged him to see the psychologist again, to get away from the Methadone, and to try harder to get himself under control. Agreeing with it all, he returned to his job and his home.

I do believe that a part of me knew that this was not the end but just another in a continuing line of episodes. I was not wrong. Scarcely a month passed and the other shoe hit the floor.

Michael got a DUI. He was driving home from work and had stopped at a grocery store and gotten a few things. At a traffic light, he went to sleep and the traffic all around him backed up. The police came and ticketed him and took him to jail. He called his brother Mark who drove up to take care of things. He got Michael out of jail and took him home where he slept for three days. He was so loaded with drugs on top of the Methadone that he was almost comatose.

While Michael was sleeping, Mark tried to clean up his apartment where it seemed that he had been quite lax. Mark stayed with him until he was on his feet and able to take care of himself at which time he came to my house and told me the entire story. I called Michael and went up to see him so that I could see for myself what was going on.

Sure enough, it was pretty bad. He had been put on leave from his job for the DUI and ordered to get help. That became my job. At length, we decided that he could not keep on like he was going. So, he took extended leave and I went up to help him put all of his things in storage and give up his apartment. I brought him and all of his clothes and things to my house and set him up in my guest room.

I made rules: he could do NO drugs or have ANY alcohol in my house; he would see a psychologist at least once a week; when he and the psychologist set up a plan for him we would keep that plan; he would help me with general housekeeping and keep his room and clothing clean and neat; he would go with me to church. His attitude was terrible. He resented having to give up his little place and he resented having rules to live by. He was aware that he had no alternative unless he could get himself clean. He could not go back to work nor have a place for himself in his present condition. So, he felt like he was in prison.

At length, the visits to the doctor and supervised living seemed to be good for him. His negatives became positives for the most part. He was looking better and certainly acting better. I had a little dog and he and that little dog became best buddies. I began to relax.

I had retired from teaching and had an online job that required me to make a trip to Washington, DC periodically. Things were going so well that I felt confident in Michael to be gone for four days and three nights. We discussed it and how he would need to take care of the dog and the house and that he was on the honor system to keep the rules just like I was there. He was totally agreeable.

So, off I went.

The next day I came back to my hotel room and had an urgent message to call home. My heart hit my feet. I was terrified. I called and sure enough things were not good.

Michael had gone to the store and gotten a milk shake, on the way back to the house, he had been so interested in the ice cream that he rear-ended a car and totaled his own vehicle doing damage to the other car as well. When the police came, he failed the breath test and got a DUI as well as the another ticket. He had gotten drugs from somewhere. Now, he knew no one in this town for I had moved about three years before. How he found someone, I do not know until this day, but he had a great supply of Xanax and was high at the time of the accident. His driver's license was suspended.

So, I came home to find that all of the work we had been doing to get him straightened out was in vain. I explained to him that he would not be able to return to work nor have his own place again until he conquered whatever had such a hold on him.

So, we started over. With no vehicle he was not able to go off by himself, so I felt sure that he was going to be unable to find another supplier. How wrong I was.

He did do better. He fell right back into the rules and with a minimum of fanfare we were getting along well. He was back with the doctor and I was pretty confident. One day he was just so antsy that he wanted to get out of the house for a bit. He made all kinds of promises and so I gave him the keys to my car and permission to go a few miles away to a restaurant to have a meal by himself. Yes, I had trepidation, but I had to trust him sometime.

This was not the time. He came in my back door about an hour later so excited. He was grinning from ear to ear telling me that he had met a girl and that they were going to go to the movies if it was alright with me. I got up to talk to him and realized that the car was not in the carport. I asked him where it was and he was stunned: he had left it running and it had rolled out of my driveway across the street into the yard of another house and down between the houses before stopping against some shrubbery. One of the houses was vacant but the other was not. Thankfully the car had not hit the house. But, as it backed out of my driveway it ran over my mailbox tearing out the suspension of the car and doing $5,000 worth of damage. I would learn later that there was no girl, he was high and wanted to get back to the guys he had met so that they could "party."

We were back to square one again.

My daughter in Texas had to have cancer surgery several months later. By that time, Michael was doing fairly well and again, I was faced with the need to leave him for a few days to go and be with her. He assured me that all was well and that he had learned his lesson. Trying to be careful, I took my car keys and hid them in the toe of a pair of shoes stored in the very top of my closet at the bottom of a stack of out-of-season shoes.

I had been in Texas for three days when my son, Mark, called to tell me that he had gotten a call from the police in a town about 150 miles away. Michael had driven my car up the interstate highway apparently going to each town seeking drugs. He had gotten to the hospital in this town and they saw what he was doing and that he was high anyway and called the police who held him until Mark could get there. The only way that they would release him was if he went straight into drug rehab—this would be his fourth stint.

I was 1,000 miles away, but Mark signed the papers and Michael was taken by the hospital personnel to rehab. My car was brought back to my house by Mark's wife who had ridden up with him for that purpose. We were all so involved in these episodes that we truly understood that it does take a village.

I quickly got myself together and convinced Charlaine to come back to Georgia with me where she could recuperate and I could take care of Michael and his "situation."

When we got to Atlanta, Mark and Michael met us at the airport. Michael had this sheepish look on his face and all that he could say was, "I'm sorry. I am so sorry." When we got home and were alone, just the two of us, he began to cry, to weep, and to heave. I saw him wracked with the most excruciating pain which was not physical, but deep down in the depths of his soul. He told me that he just wanted to die. I just wanted to weep myself. So, I did. We shared our tears.

Two days went by and he was out of it again which meant that he had to go into out-patient rehab at another facility. Charlaine was still recuperating and in a good bit of pain, but she rode with me to take him to the hospital where I checked him in for an extended stay.

All of our efforts to include him in our family life had gone awry. Christmas had always been our time to all come together and have family activities and dinner. This was very difficult with Michael. He wanted to come, but as soon as he was there he wanted to go for a ride—which we learned was code for "find some drugs." Birthday dinners were the same. We would all come to celebrate and he would be so nervous and moody. Often his language was so vulgar and his remarks so mean that the occasion was spoiled.

At Mark's wedding, he had gotten so drugged up that all he wanted to do was "go to a strip club." Of course all of us were embarrassed but we genuinely tried to make the best of the situation. The wedding was beautiful. The reception was lovely. Charlaine and I got Michael back to the hotel and into bed. When we awoke the next morning, he was gone, leaving a note that he had to be at work that evening.

At Charlaine's wedding, he had flown to Texas on the plane with my sisters who were aware of his problems. They reported that he was so anxious and unhappy that they were fearful for him. When he got to Texas, he was dressed in his most shabby clothes including a prison windbreaker that was soiled and ragged. I had instructed him what to wear and even lain out his clothing. All of my family were staying at the same hotel where Michael had a room all to himself. He holed up in that room and did not come out. For the rehearsal, he was so anxious that none of us knew what to expect. He went to the dinner, but did not eat, just scowled and begged to "get out of here." At the wedding, he was like a cardboard cutout of himself. On the plane home, my sisters reported that he was sullen and grim.

Keeping the rules was becoming more and more of a problem for him. Going to church was a nightmare. He had promised that he would go to church with me, and he would try to keep that promise; however, he would go to sleep as soon as he got still and quiet. I would nudge him to awaken him and he would get more and more angry. By the time church was over, I was a nervous wreck. He was paranoid.

We thought that perhaps if he went to Sunday School and met people his age that he would be more comfortable. So, I enlisted the help of some of the church people and we found a class of singles his age—some of them were divorced, some had never married, but all were single. He was fine with going to the class, but when it was over, he shared with me that he had gone to sleep and dropped his Bible which awakened him embarrassing him totally. He refused to go back. At church, he was sure that everyone was looking at him, so we would sit in the back. He was never comfortable. I tried and tried, but he finally got to the point he refused to go again.

He and I made a trip to visit Charlaine and her husband in Texas. What an error that was! First, he did not get along with her husband who he proclaimed to be "lame." Going out to eat was a nightmare. He never liked the place, the food was not what he was accustomed to, the people were looking at him and on and on it went. Finally, it was time to go back home. On the night before, we were deciding on what time to get up to make our flight which was very early. We decided we would have to get up about 4:30 AM. He said, "Well, I will get up and 3 AM so that I can have the bathroom for my shower and all." The little house was tight with all of us in it, so Charlaine suggested that he take his shower the night before to avoid that early hour. He blew up and of all the cursing and hateful remarks I had ever heard from him, this beat it all. Probably, I was tired and overwrought from all of the problems we had endured, but I burst into tears. She was trying to deal with him. Her husband just left. I saw no way out of it. That is how low I had sunk. I asked her to take us to a hotel where he could get up at whatever hour and do whatever he wanted and we would get on the way home at the proper time. She refused so he went ballistic again.

At length, he ran out of steam and went to bed. The next morning, he refused to shower so we went to the airport and home. All of that had just about wrecked me. When we got home, I told him frankly that something had to be done. No one could keep on living with these constant ups and downs and the almost violent outbursts. Plus, the bullying of all of us with the cursing and demeaning remarks should not continue. That made him angry and he wanted to leave, but he had no vehicle. He went into his room and broke several pictures, threw his books around and raved and ranted until he finally fell asleep. That was the moment that I knew we were not getting anywhere and none of us were getting any good out of life. I just did not know what to do.

Unfortunately, I did not have to worry about it for long. He had made friends with the couple next door to me who facilitated a lot of his dealings. I still do not understand how it all happened, but while I was at church one Sunday, they used my computer to get online and find one of those sites where all kinds of drugs can be ordered without a prescription, and found one of my credit card statements in my file and ordered a hundred Xanax for him. When I went to the mailbox and found the order, I opened it and found the pills. I was furious! I hit the ceiling. Then, I made a big mistake. Instead of flushing them down the toilet, I hid them in a box of buttons and sewing materials.

The next day, I went to the grocery and when I returned, he had found them. How, I do not know, but he did. He was high as a kite and so pleased with himself. All he could do was rale at me because he wanted to have his own place, his own car, and his own life. A part of me understood and wanted that for him as well.

Chapter Fifteen

Retirement

The latest rehab stint (this was number 6) was only for two weeks. When I picked him up he was humble, apologetic, and seemingly filled with remorse. As soon as we were in the car, he began to explain that he had not meant to disobey, but that he just "could not help it." Naturally, that was not comforting to me at all. We discussed some of the changes that would need to be made in an effort to help him conquer the addiction and live with the pain.

He was agreeable to any condition that I set forth. He would keep his room tidy, help with the housework, keep his bathroom in tip top shape and attend all of the Narcanon meetings along with some AA meetings as well. I knew that I was committing myself to a lot of additional responsibility because I would have to drive him to each meeting, wait for him, and drive him home. However, I had weighed the conditions and decided that if he could make and keep the commitment, I could too. So, we embarked on this new plan.

Then came the nightmares which were terrible!

Almost every night he would awaken me screaming and fighting the pillows. At times, he would even be up tearing at the bed and yelling obscenities. He never was able to tell me what the dreams were about, only that he was terrified. When he would become calm enough, we would go into the living room and have some hot chocolate, watch some TV, or just chat for a while as he calmed down. He was taking a medication to help him with his anxiety which was supposed to help him sleep as well. This did not work all of the time however.

Each Tuesday, I would drive him the 125 miles one way to the Methadone clinic to get his medicine. We would leave at 3 AM to be there when it opened at 5 AM. He would get the medicine and we would drive back home arriving by 7 AM. He would be miserable on the trip up, often in a fetal position in the passenger seat. After taking a dose, he would be a great mood on the way back as we stopped for breakfast. I hated those trips for I saw him at the mercy of that drug and wondered if he was really better off.

We also were driving to see his psychiatrist once a week at which time he would have a list of the questions that had arisen, the problems he had encountered, and his reactions to the medications. At one of these meetings, I was called into the office where the doctor explained that Michael's anxiety was growing and not responding to the medication, the discussions, nor the efforts Michael was supposed to be making to control those feelings. At that time, the doctor repeated what we had heard during his elementary school days, his middle school days, and his high school days, "Michael has a mental illness." He went on to say, "I don't know what will happen to him in a year, or two, or twenty. And neither do you. But I know, and you know, that this will be with him forever."

Because Michael had been with this doctor longer than any, he had a better idea of what was happening in Michael's brain as well as with his body and his emotions. As far as an explanation for why Michael was this way, there did not seem to be a way to accurately pin it down. He shared with me that Michael's premature birth and the seizure he suffered in the incubator likely had affected the final development of some of the important nerve endings in his brain which never really connected as a result. That likely played a big part in what was happening even now.

The doctor went on to cite the sexual abuse as an infant and how that may have begun the circle of abuse that continued which left Michael feeling unsafe and insecure. He went on to explain that while Michael was only four years old at the time of the second abuse, the fact that he was forced by the older boy to do something that was not comfortable for him, something that was not only out of the ordinary, but which left him feeling guilty and used. In all likelihood, those feelings had grown as Michael matured and were magnified by the guilt that he felt. This was likely the root of his resentment of authority—his guilt and insecurity increased each time he was subjected to rules and authority that enforced them.

At this time, I was brought up short and had to remember how I had worried about him all of the time when he was a baby, a toddler, going to school, playing ball, growing up. I worried about everything. I realized then that I was actually engaged in some sort of mind game, like a crossword puzzle. Life was so intricate and so fragile, especially his.

There were so many moving parts to our lives, it was impossible to anticipate what was next for him. There were simply too many factors, especially when the outside world and other people played such a huge role in his life. With his growing need for independence, there was a pitfall in overprotection. I realized that some time when we did everything right, something bad could just happen. Life is as simple and as scary as that.

There could be a case made for the fact that Michael had elected to go into law enforcement in an effort to become the authority and thereby deal with his problems. However, the terribly violent incident when he was so badly hurt in the hostage act in the prison had exploded all of the feelings that he had kept locked away and brought anew the feelings of guilt, insecurity, and danger at all turns. This had destroyed his self-esteem and any security that he had managed to build. To deal with that, he had found the release of drugs and alcohol. When he was in a stupor of either drugs or alcohol he did not have to deal with these feelings. That was the condition we were dealing with at this time.

Needless to say, I was at a loss about what my role in all of this had to be. I did not want to become his warden, but I was put into that position. My task was to do the overseeing with patience and compassion but with a strong hand at the same time.

Michael's anger problems were beginning to intensity again. He was angry that he had no car, no job, no place of his own. He resented having to "live with my mother." Every single day he would go through a litany of those issues and ask over and over why had all of this happened to him. We were still going to the Methadone Center weekly. The Methadone was supposedly keeping him from drug seeking and from alcohol. Those were terrible times. At time he would put a CD into the player and blast the heavy metal music in the car. I hated this with a passion, but was willing to endure if it brought him comfort.

When we would get to the center, he would go in and await his turn. The center opened at 5 AM and we were there when it opened each week. He would greet the other patients waiting in line with his head down, sullen, sick, and resentful of having to wait. He would pay his fees, turn in his seven empty bottles, be given a dose there and six bottles of medicine to bring home and take one a day for the week. I believe that he would visit a bit, perhaps go to the bathroom and return to the car smiling, happy, relaxed, ready to go to breakfast. I was always stunned at the remarkable difference that occurred within just minutes.

We would go to a restaurant and have breakfast. He would eat heartily even though he had not been eating for two or three days. He would laugh and be so charming that I often felt that I was in some sort of alternate dimension. On the drive back home, he would outline all of the things that we were going to do and the places that we would go. I learned to enjoy these moments knowing that they would not last.

What I learned was that Michael was not taking the methadone as he was supposed to take it—one bottle a day. Instead, he was taking two bottles a day and on occasion three. This would leave him with no medicine for the last day or so and bring on the despondency. He began to seek drugs to make up the days when he had no methadone. He had made some friends in our neighborhood and would "go for a ride" with them from time to time—running errands and the like. That is when he found his suppliers and picked up the drugs to make it through.

When I learned about this, I knew that something had to be done. Prohibiting him from going off with the friends was a part of this, but he began to take long walks which I learned took him to a nearby pharmacy where he had a forged prescription. Furious that a pharmacy was knuckling under to him, I devised a plan. I called every pharmacy in the area and described our situation. I described him, even faxed pictures to those who would accept them, and begged them not to fill ANY prescription unless I was with him. Most of them were eager to cooperate. In fact, the next time he presented himself at a pharmacy, he was turned away. That day he went to three pharmacies and none of them would accept his prescription.

While this was a victory, it brought on incredible anger. He was raving mad. He knocked over lamps, refused to eat, kicked the dog, screamed and yelled obscenities, the dog, and life in general. He was totally out of control. Repeatedly he decried his plight in life—no job, no car, no money, no place of his own, nothing that made him happy.

We were working on getting his retirement and social security in place so that he would have money and would be relieved of the underlying feeling that he was going to have to go back to work. The retirement pay would be enough for him to get a place of his own and pay some of his bills, but he needed the social security in order to be truly on his own.

When the retirement went through, he did experience some relief, but also some anxiety. He had to return his uniforms but he did not want to go to the facility and talk to the people there. So, when we went to the Methadone Clinic, we took his uniforms in two boxes and I went into the facility and returned them. They had cards, letters, and little gifts that the guards and staff had collected for him, but he would not go in. I collected them and took them out to the car. He would not even look at them. I never knew if he was so glad to have that chapter closed that he wanted no reminder, or if he was sad to see that part of his life over and felt that he would miss it. At any rate it was disconcerting and made him so uncomfortable.

That was the catalyst to new episodes of anger. He stormed through the house decrying the fact that he wanted to be on his own. He shared with me that he felt like a failure because he was having to live with me and not on his own. He wondered if his things were safe in storage and if he would ever have an apartment and a car gain. Of course, this was made more troublesome when he got his driver's license back. After more than two years, he took the class in driver's safety, and passed all of the doctor's tests to qualify for his license. That set him on fire to go back to the life that he had "enjoyed" before. Nothing that I could do would remind him that he had NOT enjoyed that life. We talked about his drinking and the drugs that had led him to forego that life. He remembered how miserable he had been at work. But, all of this just meant that he wanted to be on his own.

Michael would be fine for a while and then he would become very quiet, withdrawn and want nothing to do with anyone. The nightmares were back after some time. He would wake up screaming and sweating. The nightmares became violent. One night I tried to bring him out of one and he knocked me across the room. He shouted about an escape and a prisoner. He saw a weapon, "Was it a knife?" he screamed. He came at me and I fell to the floor. He grabbed me up and was holding me by my neck and screaming when he woke up. He looked at me startled beyond measure. His pupils were dilated and he looked around, released me, and sank to the floor weeping. He could not stop. I sat holding him for the rest of the night as he poured out his heart and described the visions he was seeing.

The doctor told me the next day that Michael had simply been unable to cope with all that had happened to him. He went on to say that he had tried to live up to what others expected of him but that the pressure grew and grew until the lid was about to blow off. He went on to tell me, "Mike has an illness. More and more doctors are coming to believe this is caused by a chemical reaction in the brain that destroys rational thought. Going on to remind me that not too many years before society had dealt with this as "demon possession." Or, the condition had been treated with ridiculous methods such as injections of horse serum, enemas, and locking the individual away. The doctor concluded that Michael's psychosis had been triggered and that he needed help because he was broken. In describing the nightmares, he said that "In the day he sees things he needs to see, but when he is asleep he sees what is really there."

How to deal with it was another matter. This doctor placed him on mood altering drugs and a sleeping medication. There were minimal results. Things were back to bad again. The medications had been only a band aid, a feeble attempt to heal a broken life. The violent nightmares returned. The violent episodes of anger returned. His displeasure at his life returned. He railed all night and all day. Wandering the house at night, he was unapologetic for his actions. Life at our home became episodes of great anger and frustration coupled with episodes of weeping and decrying mankind.

Things got so uncomfortable that I knew we could not continue like this. My son, Mark, had grown so displeased with the situation that he would not let his own son, then about six years old, to even visit me because Michael was there. We never knew how Michael would be when my grandson might come. He might have played with him or he might have been on one of his obscene rants. Mark made the choice to stay away as well. This hurt me personally. My loyalties were divided. But, Michael had no one else.

I sought the help of the psychiatrist. He told me that my only choice was to cut ties with Michael. He said that Michael's displeasure was with himself more than with me. He was needing the drugs and the alcohol and because he could not get them his anger was growing. I had not feared for my safety, but the doctor told me that I should. After much discussion, I knew that I had to make a choice. I could not discuss it with my son or my daughter because they were exhausted from handling the mood swings, the anger, the obscene behavior, and felt that things were only getting worse.

The next day was a dreadful day of shouting and incrimination. I knew that the time had come. I told him that I knew that things were not what he wanted them to be, nor were they what I wanted them to be; however, I felt that he deserved to live his life, not just to exist in the prison of my house. I told him that he was worthy of being loved and supported for the person he was, not the one that he thought he was. Then I told him that we were all going through the motions of living and that he deserved so much more than that. He was stunned and quiet for a bit. Then he started again about wanting his own place, a car, and his life back. I could only agree.

So, I prayed and prayed about it and finally made the decision to expel Michael from my home.

Chapter Sixteen

The Catalyst

The decision having been made, following through with it was the most difficult time in my life. I went to the bank and withdrew five hundred dollars. I prayed for the strength to do this and hold back my tears and my fears. That evening when Michael began his tirade loudly complaining of wanting to be independent, wanting a place of his own, and the like. I agreed with him. He was stunned.

I reminded him that he had raged about this to the point that I agreed with him. I outlined my plan: I will give you five hundred dollars; I will take you downtown where there are cabs, hotels, restaurants, and freedom; you may not come back here at night—you are on your own. Further, I told him that this would not get him an apartment, but he could find a job, a place to stay, get food to eat and be on his own until he had the funds to get an apartment. With chagrin, I told him that there was no more money, this was his seed fund, the rest was up to him.

He was delighted. He packed his bag, took the money and got into my car. I fulfilled my part of the plan. When I drove away and left him in front of a downtown hotel, my heart was breaking; however, I knew that what I was doing was for his good. This was the only way that he was going to learn. This had to be done. I had no idea how it would turn out, but I had turned it over to God and trusted Him for the results.

Three days went by.

About eight o'clock that Wednesday, I got a telephone call that Michael was in jail in a nearby county. He had sideswiped an eighteen-wheeler on the interstate highway and totaled the rental car he was driving. His bail was set at five thousand dollars. I could bring that money to them and he would be released to me or I could put up my house as collateral and he would be released. When I asked, they told me that he was not hurt but had been driving under the influence.

I was stunned. I asked, "The influence of what?" The deputy said one word, "Methadone!" My heart broke.

My instructions were to go to our local sheriff's office and he would make the arrangements to accept my house as collateral and Michael would be released. The sheriff in the county where he had the accident would see that he was driven to my house that night. So, at nine P.M., I drove downtown alone to the sheriff's office. There were all kinds of people standing around there. I was terrified. With a prayer on my lips I went in and told them of my mission. With an apology, they told me that computers were down and they could not help me for about three hours. I took one look at the surroundings and knew that I could not stand around there until midnight hoping the computers would be up and running. I went home.

The next morning, I went to my bank and withdrew five thousand dollars which meant a second mortgage on my house, drove up the interstate highway to the county where

Michael was being held. I paid the bond and waited for about two hours until they released him.

During the hours between being informed of the accident and that time, I had determined that the time for action above and beyond anything we had thought of before was now. I formulated a plan.

The judge talked to me and asked me what I was going to do about Michael. He knew the entire background and was prepared to punish him thoroughly but wanted to exercise some compassion. I shared my plan of which he approved totally. Michael was released to me with a court date.

He walked out of the door with the biggest smile on his face. He was not hurt at all; his hair was not even mussed. He had his bag with the methadone under his arm as he gave me a hug. Laughing and congenial, he told all of the officers goodbye and we went to my car.

We drove over to the wrecked rental car which had been towed to the sheriff's compound. He went through the wreckage and redeemed his bag of clothing, some CDs, and his sunglasses. As he retrieved his things, he was complaining that he only had three bottles of Methadone because "that copy must have stolen the rest of it." I just stayed quiet. I knew that I could not reason with him when he was like this. At last, he was ready to go home.

As we got onto the highway to go home, he turned to me with the biggest smile and said, "Well, that wasn't so bad was it?"

I lost it!

He had been able to rent a car, drive himself back to where he had been living, reconnect with some of his old friends, go to the Methadone Clinic, get a week's supply of medicine, stay with a friend, and had been on the road back to my house where he had a job lined up!

With a week's supply of medicine, he had taken three bottles of it—not just the one he should have taken—and was driving down the interstate when he went to pass the truck. He showed no remorse, nothing. Just, "Well, that wasn't so bad!"

I pulled off of the road onto the shoulder, and turned to him. Shaking like a leaf, I went over all that had happened. I told him how he had risked not only his life but the lives of everyone on the road. I went over the abuse of the drugs and the fact that he had spent the night in jail. Then I told him my plan.

Mark and I had investigated residential rehabilitation centers for narcotic addicts some months before. We had narrowed our choices to two Narcanon facilities—one in Oklahoma and one in Canada. Not all facilities would accept Michael because of the Methadone usage. The fee was twenty-five thousand dollars which had to be paid upon entry—the rest of my second mortgage. The patient would stay there for at least a year and until there was complete rehabilitation. Michael had been adamant that he would not go to one of these places when Mark and I had talked to him about it. At this time, I told Michael that on Sunday he was flying to Michigan where he would be admitted and there he would stay for at least a year.

He looked at me aghast refusing to even talk about it. Adamantly declaring, “NO WAY! I told him that was fine. If he did not want to go there, we would turn around and take him back to the jail where he would stay until his trial date at which time he would receive his punishment.

Again, he was stunned! He stammered and stuttered refusing to talk about it. I turned the car around to go back and he began to backtrack telling me that we would talk about it. I kept going. I was done talking.

Before we got to the jail, he grabbed my arm and said, “Okay, okay, I will go. Just take me home.”

So, I did.

Once home, he took a shower, went to bed and to sleep. I got on the phone making the arrangements with the facility. When I had cleared that hurdle, I made the flight arrangements for Sunday morning. By the time Michael awoke, everything was settled.

I gave him a list of the things he would need to pack, some of which we would have to go and purchase. The information on the facility which I had printed out, I gave to him along with the flight information. Then, I prepared lunch.

He began to beg, to make promises about what he would do, to threaten, to cajole, and to claim that no one could make him go.

I went on about my day and let him rage. That night the nightmares were terrible. I felt so sorry for him knowing that the events of the day had contributed to this, but aware that if something was not done now, we were never going to be able to fix him.

Because he had taken all of his methadone, by the second day he was in withdrawal. He was sick, sweating, unable to sleep, could not eat. This was terrible. I was in my office when he came to the door, positively green in his face, he said, "I give up. I will go."

Finally, we were making a real step forward. At least that is what I thought. So, on Sunday morning, we drove to the airport, and I saw him to his plane. He had a check for twenty-five thousand dollars, a hundred dollars in cash for spending money which the facility had requested he bring, his bag of clothes, some books, and all of the papers that had been requested. This was a direct flight and a person from the facility would meet the flight in Detroit, so the likelihood of him changing his mind, was a non-entity.

When, I saw him enter the ramp to the plane, I had no idea what would be the outcome, but I knew we had made the effort. For now, that had to be enough.

I thanked God for the strength to get this far and begged for mercy and success for Michael. Then, spent, I went home.

Chapter Seventeen

The Beginning of the End

Michael settled into the routine in Michigan quite well. He called home once a week and we chatted about every little thing. He made friends—after all, the other patients there were in the same shape as him, so he had nothing to hide. He would ask me to send him things: cigarettes, candy, books, things like that. Inquiring about the family, he wanted to keep up with everything that was happening at home. In turn, he kept me apprised of "the family" he was developing there.

I must say, I began to relax. For the first time in many years, I knew that he was safe! I did not go to sleep in fear that I would be awakened by a nightmare or a phone call about something terrible that had happened to him. Each time he called, I heard new strength and commitment to the objective we had in mind. My prayers were being answered.

I cannot say enough about the Narcanon program. They saved Michael's life. The regimen of Scientology which they espouse seemed to fit the need of which Michael was not even aware existed in his life. He ate healthy, had chores to do, and got plenty of sleep. All of the things we had striven to implement in his life were now happening.

A year went by and he came home for a visit.

Oh, my, the change in him.

He looked wonderful! He was healthy and happy. He laughed a lot, and his skin was marvelously tanned and clear. His eyes had lost that flat, dull look and now sparkled. He was a different person.

Mark came to visit and was thrilled at the results. We all felt humbled by the success that had come Michael's way. He shared some of his experiences, letting us know that he had worked very hard to achieve what we were seeing. He told us about the horrors of the "drying out" process and how he had almost died. Sharing some of the work he was doing, there was pride in his voice. We realized that not only was he now feeling safe in his world, but he regained some of the self-esteem that had eluded him for so long. He was confident and so alive. Happiness reigned supreme in our lives and in my heart.

Home for a week only, we were pleased with the results and with his plans. He shared with us that not only had he completed the program, but he had been offered a position at the facility working with the "students" as a sort of counselor. The position gave him room and board along with a salary and access to any of the counseling or other services he might feel that he needed.

The responsibility that this showed was extreme. Not only had he proven himself to the staff of the facility, but he had for the first time in his life gained the confidence to believe in himself. This was nothing short of a miracle.

So, he went back to Michigan and worked for the facility for another year. Then he came home to stay. He had reached a plateau in his healing process. He had experienced life clean and sober. He liked it. But, he was out of that climate now and he had to find a way to stabilize himself.

In the time that he was away, there had been a refusal by the Social Security Administration to grant him a disability even though all of his doctors and the people with whom he had worked had furnished statements and the like. On his behalf, we had secured an attorney who managed to get a hearing with the judge and a rehabilitation counselor. Because Michael was away, I had been requested to come to the hearing. This was our last chance to get a disability for Michael which would enable him to be on his own when he came back home.

In a nervous dither, I sat in the judge's chambers and heard Michael's case presented. The rehabilitation counselor had prepared a presentation on jobs for which Michael might be qualified rather than going on disability. To my absolute amazement, the judge declared that the situation with which Michael had been forced to deal in the prison qualified him for consideration. Further, he stated that the business with Michael's resentment of authority spoke to the horror he had been forced to endure. With all of this information, he granted Michael one hundred per cent disability with back pay to the time of his retirement. Our prayers had been answered.

A neighbor had a beautiful Acura car that he was selling. Michael's settlement to retire had left him with a hefty sum in his bank account and he wanted to buy the car. So, Michael came home some months later knowing that he would have an apartment, a car, a life of his own. Certainly that contributed to his positive attitude.

We set about finding an apartment for him. This was actually an easy task because he was so happy at the possibility that most anything would have pleased him. But he chose a relatively new apartment complex where he selected a two-bedroom apartment within walking distance of shops and restaurants. We were told that most of the residents were about his age and that there would be plenty of opportunities to make friends around the pool and in the club house.

So we contracted a moving van and went back to the town where Michael had lived and collected his things from storage. He realized that all of the fuss and furor he had caused about his things not being safe had been in vain. It was all there. His new attitude however had him looking askance at his possessions. He decided that he did not want to begin his new life with most of these things, so he made a gift of his living room furniture, his washer and dryer, and a few other things to the moving men. He moved his stereo, CDs and records, his books, and other possessions into the new place and went out and bought new living room furniture and a new washer and dryer. His bedroom suite was new when he got sick, so he kept it but got a new mattress and box springs along with a new TV and DVD player.

He was all set. That plateau became a comfortable place for him. He had his cell phone and all of his friends on speed dial. All of his dreams had come true. He sat down and took inventory and realized he was on his own.

While he had no job, he had a regular income from his disability. In short, the things that had caused him the most angst were now his. All of the doctors and counselors had agreed that he was not ready to work, and indeed might never be able to hold a steady job. He just needed to go one day at a time.

So, all of us took a deep breath and relaxed confident that this was the best thing in the world for Michael and that all was going to be well. He was stabilized but he was not making much progress.

Chapter Eighteen

The End

Well, it was pretty wonderful for a while. He made friends, visited with us, and set about establishing a new life for himself.

Unfortunately, as had been the case most of his life, Michael was not careful in the choices of friends. Some of the people who were befriended by him were not the best of choices. Before too long, he was buying beer and having a blast with some of the people he had met there.

He moved one of these new acquaintances in as his roommate. The young man had access to drugs without having to get a forged prescription and go to a pharmacy and before too long, we were suspicious that Michael was back using drugs. He spent more and more of his time closeted away in that apartment.

He came to my house once with broken ribs, a black eye, and several cuts and scrapes. Shocked, I questioned his appearance, whereupon he told me that he and been playing football with some kids in the area and fell onto a curb. I did not believe it for one moment, but I was dealing with a grown man who became quite annoyed when I questioned further. Much later I would learn that these and other injuries came from the roommate!

My son, Mark, had been selected by the SSA to be Michael's guardian of finances, meaning that he had access to Michael's accounts, paid all of Michael's bills, and gave him a weekly allowance. This proved to be one of the best things that could have happened.

Michael was so eager to have friends and to be liked by people that his money went as soon as it was received. He bought food for his friends, gambled with them, bought beer for them and drank with them. The roommate paid no rent but enjoyed the food and drink as well as the hospitality.

No matter how we tried to talk to Michael and show him what was happening, it meant nothing. He refused to admit that his so-called friends were using him. He made friends with the people upstairs—a single mother with two children. He wound up buying groceries for them. She wound up visiting Michael and spending the night. He did admit that they were having sex, much to my chagrin.

Mark was having all kinds of difficulties with Michael and his money. Michael would get his allowance and within two days have no money. He would call Mark begging for money so that he could eat. Of course, it was Michael's money, but Mark was charged with seeing that is was spent appropriately. The two of them had many, many arguments over all of this.

Michael's apartment became a flop house for all of his so-called friends. The roommate he had befriended was arrested for drugs and Michael was back on his own for a while. Unfortunately, it was only for a while. Soon there was another young man staying in his guest room. He assured us that this was a "good guy" with a college education and a good job We would later learn that the young man actually had neither, he just talked a good game.

The people with whom Michael had been in treatment in Michigan began to call him as well. Michael literally lived on his cell phone. I think that every one of the patients in Michigan had and used his phone number. Some of them called out of friendship and they would chat about what they were doing now and how they were or were not doing. Michael would come away from some of those conversations thankful for all that he had when some of his friends had gone home to families that turned them away and consequently had nothing.

Some of those friends called wanting money. The word seemed to get out that Michael had his own place, car and the like, so they knew that he was a good guy and sure enough, Mark would get a call for money to send to these people all across the country. Of course, none of the money was ever paid back.

Then, some of them wanted a place to stay. One girl called and begged for a place to stay until she could get a job in a nearby community. She came, with her drugs, and stayed for a week while they both got and stayed high. When Michael's money ran out, she left.

So it was that Michael's good nature got him in even more trouble. The people in the apartment complex knew that he was an easy touch and shared their drugs or sold some to him. He had tried the pharmacies with genuine prescriptions from a doctor who was later arrested for writing so many painkiller prescriptions. No pharmacy would fill one for Michael. His friends, however, shared with him—for a price.

Mark fought the good fight. He would deny Michael extra funds until he could no longer bear the begging and threatening. Michael made all kinds of trouble for Mark and his family. At all hours, Michael would call for Mark to bring him money and there would ensue the refusal and the repeat calls. At other times, Michael would have a friend drive him to Mark's house—no matter that they were having dinner, or that Mark's son was doing homework. There would then ensue the argument in person. The "friends" would coach Michael about what to say. They would convince him that Mark was just being mean, or even that Mark was using all of Michael's money for his own purposes. That was really difficult for Mark when he was simply doing what he was charged to do and what was best for Michael.

We all realized that Michael was on a downward spiral again and that we needed to do something about it before he sank so low that recovery was impossible. But, what to do? Talking did not good, he disputed everything that we said. He was constantly surrounded by the people who were benefiting from his condition and making him feel that Mark was his enemy and that we were all prying.

The good times vanished. The times when we could visit him in his apartment and watch a movie or have a meal were over. When I did go there, the place was in such a state that I wanted to weep. Michael's own room was a shambles with clothes and books piled in the corners. Dust was everywhere, the bathroom was a nightmare. This from the guy that had been so happy to have his own place that he had dusted several times a day. What to do?

By this time, I had retired again and moved to the mountains. I kept up with Michael through Mark and through regular phone calls with him. He would call me to chat or to share some tidbit of news and I knew that things were not well, but as long as the lines of communication were open, then there was hope.

On Sundays he would call and we would watch a Falcon game together. We would cheer and lament and dissect the plays just as if we were in the room together. I could tell that about midway through the game he got looser and looser, so I knew that he was drinking. I kept the tone light as I let him know that I knew what was happening.

When he and Mark would have an argument over the money and Michael's spending, he would call me and rale about Mark and how "tight" he was. Listening to his "friends" again about Mark using his money, he broached this with me. I was furious that he would listen to people talk like that about Mark who was enduring all of the work involved with helping Michael make a go of things. So, Michael backed off.

While all of this was going on, Jackson--Mark's son, my grandson, Michael's nephew—was growing up. At his graduation from Elementary to Middle School, Michael was to go with me. I was dressed and ready and urging Michael to get ready as well. He disappeared and the time came for Mark to pick us up. I was so hurt for Mark and his family when Michael simply did not come back, instead, we saw him coming up out of the woods with the man across the hall who we were pretty sure was supplying Michael with some of his pills. Jackson had no idea, but was sad that his Uncle Mike would not be there.

Michael was rarely there for Jackson—no ballgames, no school activities, nothing. One night, Mark took Jackson to Atlanta to a Braves' game. Of course, as the game got underway, there was a call from Michael. He was at a hospital seeking drugs and the police were holding him. Mark had to leave the game, take Jackson home, and then drive back to deal with the situation. Poor Jackson never realized what was happening.

Later, after Michigan and the aftermath, when he was in his teens, Jackson realized what had been going on for all of his life. Recently, we were talking about drugs and alcohol in the schools and among young people his age and he said to me, "Grammie, after seeing all that Uncle Mike went through, I am not touching that stuff." I thought how great it was that perhaps Michael's life did mean something after all.

After one of the heated arguments with Mark in the presence of his friends, we learned that he had admitted himself to a residence rehabilitation program This gave us cause for hope. If he saw his situation as spiraling downward and took this step, then he wanted to help himself. We rejoiced and cooperated fully with this.

We had no way of knowing what the outcome of this rehab experience would be.

Michael met two girls in this rehab experience. They were from a small town not too far away. He was thrilled that they had given him their number so that they could stay in touch. He told me that he was going to call one of them whom he really liked and they were going to a movie. I got excited for him.

A few days later, he told me that the one of them was coming to see him and that they were going to go out for supper and perhaps to a movie. I thought how great it would be if Michael began to have a real life and how great it would be that he would not be so determined to hang around with the more disreputable people he had always seemed to find.

The date went well. She had driven in and met him at the theater. They went to the show and then out for dinner. They had stayed in the restaurant talking until the place closed and then she drove back home. He was happy and said that they were going out again soon. I spoke with him and he described her and how much fun they had along with his excitement at seeing her again.

Well, they did get together again, but not like he had planned.

The next that I heard was the dreaded telephone call telling me that Michael was dead.

Chapter Nineteen

Aftermath

The roommate shared that he had plans and had left the apartment at nine A.M. on Sunday after Michael had told him that the two girls had "scored some methadone" and were coming to see him and they were "going to have some fun." So, the roommate left and did not come home until about nine P.M. that night to an apartment that was dark. Calling out for Michael, he went into Michael's bedroom where he found him lying face down on the bed. Thinking that he was asleep, he touched him to awaken him when he realized that Michael was cold. At that point he called the police and then he called me.

Hysterical and two hundred miles away, I demanded that he call Mark who straightway came to the apartment arriving just as the police arrived. Mark confirmed that Michael looked like he was sleeping.

The Medical Examiner's report showed that Michael died of "Methadone Toxicity."

On the refrigerator was a slip of paper with the name and phone number of the girl who had been at the apartment that day. The police checked with her whereupon she told them that he was fine when she left.

We planned a small memorial to Michael where his aunts, uncle, and cousins came to pay respects. Charlaine flew in from Texas distraught with grief at the loss of her buddy, her brother, her partner-in-so many crimes. Also attending were a great many of Michael's neighbors and friends from the apartment complex. They came with their stories of how much they had loved him, how he had helped them, the good times that they had shared.

And, there was Jeff, Michael's childhood friend with whom he had stayed friends until the bitter end.

After the memorial, Mark and his family, Charlaine and I sat down in Mark's den and wondered what could have been done differently, what had taken his life so young, and caused him so much pain?

There is no answer.

We all agreed that Michael is in a better place today. He is not in any pain. There are no feelings of desperation, despondency, or anxiety. He is free.

How, I wish that he could have found that freedom in the goodness of life and enjoyed all of the gifts God had given him.

In the long dark nights, when sleep evades me and my thoughts inevitably go to Michael, I see him as he was as a toddler—happy, smiling, friendly, active, and loving. That is the picture that I hold in my heart. However, my soul cries out in pain because I know deep down the anxious pain that propelled him all of his teen and adult life. I still shed tears for what might have been. But, I thank God every single solitary day for taking my son home to heaven where there is no pain nor anxiety and where he can relax in the arms of his savior and God. Then, I sleep.

Chapter Twenty

What Happened

After five years, my love for Michael is still deep and real. He was a beautiful person; but, something happened to take away that happy, grinning little boy and leave a broken man who was aggressive to the point of violence, lonely and troubled with no self-esteem, never feeling safe or secure, unable to cope with the most minute tasks of daily living and "coloring within the lines." Watching him for the forty-nine years of his life, experiencing the high highs and the lowest of lows, talking with doctors, psychologists, psychiatrists, counselors and other experts, in the long, dark nights of my soul, I still ask, "What happened?"

Was it genetic?

Various doctors told us that there was a genetic disposition to addiction and depression in Michael's life. When we heard that we always despaired because we could not deliver him from that burden.

In fact, the truth is that Michael's biological parents were very young: she was sixteen and he was seventeen. Both of them were heavily into drugs and alcohol. His father had quit going to school at age fifteen because he had trouble learning: by that time, he was a veteran drug user. So, by the time he fathered Michael he was heavily into drugs and had also become addicted to alcohol. Michael's mother was still in school when she became pregnant, but was irregular in her attendance because of her heavy drug use.

The situation in their respective homes was not good either. She delivered Michael in her home town, but because she wanted to "keep him" she was sent to another state to live with her grandmother and finish school. She enrolled in school but got back into drugs so badly that she elected to give her baby up for adoption so that she could get out of her grandmother's house.

So, at three months of age, Michael was surrendered to the state agency and offered for adoption. After three months of being shuffled to foster homes, he came to live with us.

Therefore, a case can be made that Michael could have been genetically disposed to the addictions that haunted his life, and could have played a big part in the battles he fought.

Was it trauma?

More than one psychiatrist and/or psychologist told us that suffering significant trauma can cause the brain to respond differently to triggers. They cited Post Traumatic Stress Disorder (PTSD) as the definition of this condition. One doctor explained it as a "wound to the psyche", another as a reprogramming of the brain.

Michael had struggled with the question of identity for most of his life. PTSD is a profound blow to one's sense of self—to his value system, and to his belief that he can control his life. There seemed to be an emotional numbness in his life, like he did not feel entitled to experience happiness. Instead he seemed to have a hopelessness and inability to express difficult thoughts or feelings. He seemed to be his own enemy and all of his defenses were shattered. His every waking hour he was hypervigilant, extremely anxious, feared confinement and experienced an inability to communicate his feelings, chronic sleeplessness and chronic nightmares.

Michael was placed for adoption at the age of three months during which time he lived with his teenage mother and her grandmother. Upon his surrender, the agency sought an "appropriate home" for him. During the ensuring three months, he was in five different foster homes having been removed from two of them because of inadequate care, one for cruelty, and one for sexual abuse.

At that time, science was holding that environment was the great shaper of human nature. Then, more research seemed to indicate that babies were born with distinct personalities. This could explain why some children are so gregarious, others so quiet, some so crabby and others so calm. Now, science holds that this is right too that we are hardwired from the beginning. Environment can temper it, but that nature is still there.

Certainly being in a home where he was treated with cruelty would qualify as a "traumatic" event. But, following that with placement in a home where he suffered sexual abuse as an infant would qualify as well. We had no way of knowing what types of abuse he endured. He was born in another state and those records were not available to us. We did have the hospital records of the incubator incident.

In addition, he was born prematurely at a weight of four pounds and 7 ounces. While in the incubator, he suffered a “major seizure” for which he was treated with “massive doses of calcium.” We were told when we adopted him that he would likely have some sort of “condition” as a result of this and that we should “watch” him.

The pediatrician who treated Michael from the time he came to us at six months of age until he was almost six years old had these records and was aware of all that had happened. When Michael began to bite other students and become wildly active, this doctor told us that we might have a problem but that he could outgrow it. At that time, doctors did not hand out the diagnosis of hyperactivity and attention deficient disorder with the appropriate drugs as they do today. Chances are that this was our warning sign and if so trauma certainly played a part in his problem.

Certainly when you add to this the sexual experience when he was four years old, there is evidence of trauma. Of significance in this instance is the fact that he was old enough to know that this was wrong. He had been toilet trained; he knew the purpose of his body parts; he had a little brother whose private parts had never interested him. In addition, he was threatened that if he told anyone what had happened that his baby brother would be harmed. That alone told him that what happened was wrong.

Of particular interest in this incident is that Michael either could not or did not share the incident for almost forty-five years. He carried the memory of the incident and the guilt that he felt as a result of it from the time he was a little boy through puberty, teen years, into adulthood. When he finally did tell me, I was so shocked. He could not remember the boy's name, but he described him even to what he was wearing, how his hair was cut and what type underwear he was wearing. I recognized the boy immediately and even remembered the day for a group of ladies from our church were joining me for Bible study and my neighbor volunteered her twelve-year-old son to play with Michael while they were there. I carry guilt for that myself even to this day. I looked that boy up on the internet. He is a grown man now with children of his own and a very successful career. I cannot help but wonder, "Does he remember that day?"

Imagine carrying this guilt what must have gone through Michael's mind when as a twenty-one-year-old freshman prison guard assigned to death row where he was taken hostage in a stairwell and raped by a prisoner incarcerated for multiple hundred year sentences then released to be ridiculed by the other death row prisoners and even the other guards themselves. My blood runs cold to think of it.

That experience sent him to the hospital only to return to the same prison and the same area where he had to look at that prisoner every day that he worked. That was when he really began to partake of alcohol and, as I learned many years later, hard drugs as well. He even went so far as to tell me when he was about forty that all he wanted was to "forget and to be left alone."

Quite possibly these events explain some of the reasons that Michael was never able to sustain a relationship with a woman. He did not date a lot in high school—only for prom until he was a senior. Then in college he began to see girls for a while and then move on. There was no real relationship. He met another girl while in rehab and they began to see one another after they were released. Michael got a transfer to a facility near her and they moved in together. This lasted for about two years and was his ONLY relationship. That relationship had its ups and downs and was severely affected by Michael's lack of self-esteem. Everything else was fleeting at best.

-

One of the doctors even went so far as to describe combat stress and how it caused PTSD. He told us that Michael's volatility, his self-medication, withdrawal from family and friends, and his outbursts of anger were all indicators, as well as his withdrawal from sex.

Quite often, he would remark how he wished that he had what Mark had a family and a home of his own. He declared that if he ever found a girl like his sister or his sister-in-law that he was going to marry her immediately. That never happened.

Then we learned that research showed that some people are predisposed to PTSD. Some analysts think that childhood experiences likely create a heightened vulnerability. Others believe that other variables can help account for some, but not most of the occurrences of PTSD. Michael had more than his share of traumatic experiences.

So there is a lot to say for trauma playing a big part in the quality of life Mike had. He was treated with all kinds of anti-depressants and the like, but nothing gave him that security that he so greatly needed.

Was it his home life?

Many books that we read and authorities whom we consulted posed the possibility that Michael's home life and relationship with his family contributed to his problem. Of course that was a difficult pill to swallow. When we asked God to give us a child, we dedicated ourselves to that child, to giving him a happy and secure home with lots of love and acceptance and as many advantages as possible. We felt that we had been true to those commitments. Then to have to face the fact that perhaps the home we had provided, the family that we had given him was a part of the problem was difficult. But, in taking an honest look at our situation, there is much to be said for this.

Some people experience bad things as children and apparently just forget them. Others experience bad things and they stay with them for all of their lives. Some people carry their childhood memories into adulthood and wonder how the people they loved the most could do things that seemed to void all of that love. They drag their past along with them into whatever new life experience they encounter. Unable to admit the pain of the past, they move on to more and more painful experiences because they feel that they do not deserve love and happiness. Michael may well have been one of those people. We offered him a home and all of our love, support, and understanding, but obviously, it was not enough.

First, life in the ministry is like living in a fishbowl. The very house in which we lived was the property of the church.

We could not change the color of paint in the rooms or anything like that. Michael was taught from the moment he could walk to be careful not to damage the house. The yard was a part of the fish bowl and his toys and playtimes were on display and available for judgment. He was taken to church more than most children (all three of our children remember that). Some children thrive spiritually in that environment; others learn to dislike the church. He sat through adult meetings with a few toys and a book and the admonition to be perfectly quiet and still. In all of his classes, the teachers expected him to know the Bible because he was the preacher's son.

His activities in the community and at school were closely watched and judged because of who his father was. If boys his age got in trouble, the assumption was that he was a part of it and we got the call. How his hair was cut, the clothes he wore, the way he drove his van, the company that he kept, the participation in community activities was all judged far more harshly than were other boys his age.

Then, we moved a great deal. He attended four different schools by the time he graduated from high school. When he was in elementary school the system of which he was a part was forcefully racially integrated which created some degree of chaos. Most of his church friends were removed from the public schools and sent to private schools. We kept our boys in public school. That created some disturbance because the boys with whom he had been friends for some time were no longer friendly to him. After a few years, the emotional climate of the community changed and all was well again. But, perhaps the damage was done. But, the frequent moves did take a toll, I am sure. It meant a change of physical security—sometime he had his own room, other times he had to share a room. He also had to make new friends and get a reading on the people in the new community and church. This helped the other two children to adapt to other people and situations in their adult lives, but it seemed a hindrance to Michael so much so that he elected to stay in the same community where he had graduated high school and gone to college when he went to work. He did not like change.

Then our counselors talked about his relationships with parents. There was a distinct difference in his relationship with his father and his relationship me.

Charles was a demanding father. He had very strict rules and expected total compliance. Some of his rules were a bit severe and the punishment for breaking them was equally severe. He believed in corporal punishment and did not hesitate to carry it out on both of the boys. His instrument of choice when carrying out the punishment was a brush with a handle about two-and-a-half feet long and about three inches wide and half an inch thick. He wielded it with strength too. Michael was often left with broad welts on his back and bottom. Michael was a male and likely felt that he should measure up to his father. With the ambivalent relationship between Charles and Michael, there was often no one else to emulate. Charles had set expectations without providing the warmth that Michael craved.

In addition, Charles was very critical of the children. He expected Michael to "be a man" from the time he learned to walk. Tears were not permitted. He was critical of everything that Michael said and did. (He was like that with all three of the children.) Michael had a God-given talent with drawing. He was truly and artist. That is what got him a scholarship to college—he was that good. He did the cover for my first book and did artwork for the church and when he got into high school he was called upon by the school for all kinds of projects from murals to posters to logos. Charles hated that. It was not "manly" enough. When Michael would complete a project, Charles always made it a point to find something wrong with it.

When Charles was dying, it was Michael who took him to his chemo treatments and cared for him during the day. Sometime after Charles's death, Michael asked me, "Do you think that Daddy knew that I loved him?" During that discussion he said, "I don't think I ever pleased him, did I?" So, did that have a part in Michael's lack of self-esteem.

Then, there is me. Was I too far the opposite of Charles? Was I an enabler? I tried to keep a good attitude with the children. Of course, Michael did things of which I did not approve, things that I disliked, and things that disappointed me. Rather than criticize and deride him, I tried to talk to him and show him why I had the feelings that I did and tell him how things could have been done differently. I gave him second chances. Early in his life, I knew that things were different for him. I did not know why nor what to do, but I tried to find out so that we could fix it. I am a notorious "fixer." I sought books and advice from reputable sources. I tried to put into practice things that would help his confidence and enhance his self-esteem. As a result, I was constantly told that I was too soft on him, that I was making him into a sissy, making him too dependent. So, I may have been a part of Michael's problem rather than a solution. I had always tried to be what I felt that a mother needed to be: sound of mind, wholesome, healthy, good, unafraid, able to deal with the world and to thrive in any culture. Having an integrated personality would make me a well-adjusted person, I thought. But, perhaps I had missed something really important.

We were all aware that the difference in the boys' security and self-esteem were gigantic. Mark was quiet and a thinker from the time he was tiny. When he was in about the sixth grade his self-assurance and leadership began to show itself and he entered Middle School as a popular boy with both students and teachers. The church people loved him. He excelled in everything he did—sports, activities, church, and school. Michael saw all of that and resented it. He was great at football and art—diametrically opposed in many ways of thinking—but unable or unwilling to put himself out there and do what Mark did. Did that contribute?

When Charlaine came along, as the only girl of course she was different. She always had her own room and was not subjected to punishment and the like as the boys were. By the time that she was three, she was into music and playing the piano. She had friends—her peers as well as adults. She was unafraid to try anything. Her talent manifested itself and took her far. Michael could see that and often resented her ease with people and the recognition she received. Perhaps that contributed.

There was never a great deal of money in our home. Part of the ministry is that one is never in danger of getting rich. Michael never seemed to mind that as much as Mark and Charlaine. He was alright with wearing no-name jeans and the like. (Of course, Mark got the hand-me-downs, so that may have been a part of his problem.) Not until he was an adult, when he came home on Workman's Compensation did he begin to ask for money and call attention to the fact that there was never enough. He was terrible at keeping up with his own money. He was paid every two weeks and by the beginning of the second week he never had money. He would come to me at school or at home begging for money. At length, Mark took over managing Michael's money and that lasted until his death. Michael was given an "allowance" which was generous anyway it was measured, but he was always without money. Of course, we learned where the money was going—to drugs and dealers and friends—but there was no way we could get him to be responsible. Money may have been a factor as well.

So, when all of these factors are considered, perhaps our family/home life was a factor as well. I even asked a psychiatrist how Mark and Charlaine could be so different when the three of them were reared by the same people in the same circumstances. His reply was—genetics. I do pray that we were good to him because we did love him. Sometimes, children can get more attention because they seem to be in more need of attention. And then, there are children who seem so self-possessed and competent that they seem to need less. I suppose that may have been part of Michael's problem. He needed more because he did not feel safe nor secure while Mark and Charlaine felt competent in their world.

Was it rock music?

As a teenager, he exhibited a love for music. That love grew and grew. He listened to all music but gradually came to prefer rock and roll music and had his favorite artists. We learned to buy him records or give him gift certificates for records whenever there was a gifting occasion. He cherished his records.

His stereo system was not the greatest—Santa had brought it to Mark and him years ago. So, for Christmas, Santa brought him his own fairly good system which he dearly loved. But the system he enjoyed the most was the one in the little blue van. He upgraded it constantly and worked on it regularly. He would ride around the area just so he could listen to his music. Often, he would just go out to the garage and sit in the van with the music going. Years later, when he got his first real job, he bought his own stereo components with a handsome cabinet to house them and it became his prize. He learned many of the lyrics and he and I discussed them as if they were poetry.

When he realized that we were not going to have problems with his music, he was thrilled. He began to draw illustrations of the lyrics so that they looked like album covers. Music became the strongest force in his life.

.

When he and Mark were about eight and ten years old, they heard Three Dog Night do "Jeremiah Was a Bullfrog" and were smitten. We bought the record and they played that song over and over while they jumped on the beds and rolled around the room. Charlaine even got in on the act although she was only three or four. I suppose that was where Michael felt the beginnings of the love for music.

From his teens onward, his favorite group was Blue Oyster Cult. He knew each of the artists by name, where they were from how they had gotten into music and the like. True to his form, he had all of their records and played their music almost constantly. Years later when I would be driving him to his doctor appointments, he would bring his CD and play their music on the trip.

When they were chosen for membership in the Rock and Roll Hall of Fame, I could only think about how pleased Michael would have been. He felt that he was their number one fan.

His favorite song, or at least the one he referenced the most was entitled "Don't Fear the Reaper" which is a song about death. Summing up the lyrics one learns that we all come to this earth, we live, we love, and we die. There is no reason to dread it, it will come, so we should not dread (fear) it but we should embrace today. I saw no reason to ban this song, in fact, I could see some of our culture in it. Live for today, let tomorrow take care of itself seemed to mirror the lyrics. I did have a talk with Michael about setting goals and realizing that there is more to life than just today and certainly more than just "love" no matter what connotation one gives the word. He insisted that it was a "great song" and loved the music. I really cannot see that his fondness for this type of music could have infiltrated his mind to the point of causing aggression, self-loathing, and loss of security.

As an adult we were discussing them one day and I went on the web where I found their site. He was thrilled. He ordered a shirt and copied down all of their information. He was like a little kid. He wound up finding more about them and eventually called them by phone and actually talked to one of them. The guy was most impressed that Michael was so passionate about their music and they talked several times. He invited Michael backstage when they next came to Georgia. Needless to say, Michael was more than pleased.

As time went by and vinyl records were replaced by 8-track tapes, Michael made the move buying the tape for each of his records. Then, when cassette tapes replaced the 8-track, Michael redid his collection again. Finally, the cassette was replaced by the CD and there was another replacement. In the last days of his life, Michael was still adding to his treasured collections.

Something Else

We truly believed that we had tried it all. We had given him a supportive home environment, tutoring, changed school environments, fought against the bad companions. We did so much to get him away from the people who influenced him, those who drew him toward alcohol, flirtation with drugs, and even briefly an interest in the occult. But, perhaps we had alienated him and hacked away at his self-esteem. Maybe it was not his companions. Maybe it was his own spiraling depression as he tried so hard to search for answers as to what had happened to him. He certainly believed that he was of no value and kept spiraling always downward. When we felt that he was getting better, we realized that all he was doing was internalizing the torture he was enduring all alone. We were amazed at his memorial how many of those "bad companions" showed up to pay their respects. They spoke to us of his wisdom and good nature. They told us of the times he had helped them when they had nowhere to turn. And they told us about how hard he tried to make his own life better as well as theirs. They told us stories of his heartbreak and suffering.

The hard knot of emotion that surrounded my soul twisted tighter as I saw my child aggrieved and angry, not at the world or at us, but at himself. He had been bitter at his life and the results he thought he saw. He had such a tough time, and still maintained a warmth toward these people. He just did not believe that he deserved to have anyone really care about him. And, that made me so sad.

In Memoriam

In thinking back over my life with Michael, I remember the good times: when he learned to walk, seeing him in his wading pool as a toddler, watching him play football, seeing the glow on his face when we praised his artwork, the sweet goodness when he dealt with his brother and sister, the gentleness with his dying father, and the devilish grin when he teased one of us. I remember with tears in my eyes for this was my firstborn, the son of whom I had dreamed, and I loved him from the beginning and I cherish him this day.

Each year when I would teach Shakespeare, I would come to a passage from *Macbeth* that made me think of Michael. It goes like this: "The mind, the heart, and the soul. 'Canst thou not minister to a mind diseased? Pluck from the memory a rooted sorrow. Raze out the written troubles of the brain and with some sweet oblivious antidote cleanse the stuff'd bosom of that perilous stuff which weighs upon the heart.' He'd lifted his gaze from his drink as she'd spoken. Her voice remained quiet, but he'd stopped hearing the juke, the clatter, the laughter."

Then, I think again, that if only medical science had the knowledge then that they do today, might things have been different for Michael. Maybe they could have helped him as a little boy and forestalled the terror of his adolescence and adulthood. But, that does no good.

Wiping a tear, I am reminded of a thought from one of Michael's favorite books. The best way to summarize his troubles in life, his anger, his violent tendencies, his addiction, his illness, his tenderness for those whom he loved is simply to say that, Michael's life resembles the nursery rhyme he learned as a little boy.

Humpty Dumpty sat on a wall.
Humpty Dumpty had a great fall
And all the king's horses and all the king's men
Couldn't put Humpty together again.

When Michael's life was broken as a little boy, no matter who tried what, we were never able to put it back together again. He tried: with doctors, medication, training, prayer, and the obedience that came so hard to him, he did try. However, nothing that he did, or we did could fix that broken life until that fateful Sunday when he could not avoid the temptation of drugs gotten illegally, and his life on this earth, as stressful, angst-ridden and painful as it was, ended and he went to something better where we are promised peace and happiness.

I pray that on the other side, there in heaven, Michael, has found his other self and is experiencing the joy he so wanted while here on this earth. From the time that he came to us as an infant until the time he left us as an adult, my prayer has been for him to find what would make him happy. Now, I believe that he has.

Michael's life was not in vain. He taught us patience and he taught us to seek the whys and the wherefores, and to take nothing, nothing at all at face value, and to be strong in the broken places.

Acknowledgements

My grateful admiration goes to my other two children, Mark and Charlaine who lived their entire lives alongside Michael. They saw and shared his pain, counseled him, berated him, helped when he was down, and rejoiced when he was up. Neither of them ever had a good understanding of what was going on in his life. They never stopped loving him. Their fears for him often left them terrified, their passion for him to mend his broken life never waned. Their tears at losing him displayed grief in what could have been and the hope of what can be. Michael loved them dearly and was so proud of them. Their sibling bond was never broken—stretched but not broken. God bless them!

Then, I acknowledge my daughter in law, Jill—Mark's wife—who came into our family aware that Michael was broken and worked tirelessly to help him in any way possible. She sat with him when he raged, drove him when he was grief-stricken, counseled him when he needed it, and always loved him like a sister. He loved her.

Mark and Jill's son, Jackson, played a big part in Michael's life. Michael was so proud of him and predicted that he would be a "GREAT baseball player and make lots and lots of money." Jackson loved his Uncle Mike, never really understood him, but loved him. I have a picture of Mike asleep on the sofa with Jackson sleeping soundly in his arms. I treasure that.

There are many others: Jeff Sikes who was Michael's friend from their tenth grade year in high school until the day Mike died; Bob Swatko who stood beside him so many times and prayed for him always; the staff at Michigan's Narcanon who gave him back to us for five wonderful years; the many doctors who tried so hard over the years; and, his teachers who never quite understood but tried so hard to help him. I give you all my undying appreciation.

References Consulted

Adams.Tiate. 2013. *The Painkiller Addiction Epidemic, Heroin Addiction and the Way Out.* Rapid Response Press.

Conyers, Beverly. 2009. *Addict in the Family: Stories of Loss, Hope and Recovery.* Hazeldon.

Cook, Alicia. (Feb. 12, 2016) I loved a Drug Addict and Got the Dreaded Call. USA Today.

Hari, Johann. 2015. *Chasing the Scream: The First and Last Days of the War on Drugs.* USA: Bloomsbury.

Herzanek, Joe. 2010. *Why Don't The Just Quit?* Changing Lives Foundation.

How Drugs Affect the Brain. (Jan 30, 2002). MentalHelp.net.

National Institute of Drug Abuse. "Drug Facts: Understanding Drug Abuse and Addiction." Nov. 2012.R

Saving Lives from Addiction. (2003) Narconon.

The Economic Impact of Illicit Drug Use on American Society. (2011) Washington: United States Department of Justice.

Why Your Addict Will Always Choose Drugs Over Love. Jul 28, 2009. Klein Treatment Ctr.

I hope that you understand a little better the agony that an addict and his family endure for the sake of the addiction. If you do, then my job is done. Do not hesitate to contact me with comments or concerns. I love hearing from you

On Facebook, I can be found at Read My Books!

Follow me on Twitter, # Patricia S Burgess

Send me Email: http:ww.grendelb@windstream.net

My website is: http:www.patriciasuttonburgessauthor where you can follow my blog.

Other books by Patricia Sutton Burgess

Another Life

My Name Is Ruth

From the Beginning

www.ingramcontent.com/pod-product-compliance
Lightning Source LLC
Chambersburg PA
CBHW051907170526
45168CB00001B/281

* 9 7 8 1 5 1 7 3 4 4 9 9 3 *